As Jesus Cared for Women

Restoring Women Then and Now

W. David Hager, M.D.

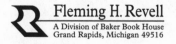

Fleming H. Revell
A Division of Baker Book House
Grand Rapids, Michigan 49516

Published by Fleming H. Revell
a division of Baker Book House Company
P.O. Box 6287, Grand Rapids, MI 49516-6287

Printed in the United States of America

Library of Congress Cataloging-in-Publication Data

Hager, W. David (William David), 1946–
     As Jesus cared for women : restoring women then and now / W.
David Hager.
          p.   cm.
     ISBN 0-8007-1751-1
     1. Women—Religious life. 2. Spiritual healing—Case studies. I.
Title.
BV4527.H34   1998
261.8'344—dc21   97-48595

All names of persons whose stories are shared have been changed to protect their privacy.

Because this book deals with women and Jesus, the female pronoun is frequently used rather than "he or she."

For current information about all releases from Baker Book House, visit
our web site:
                         http://www.bakerbooks.com

As Jesus Cared for Women

Other books by Dr. Hager

Stress and the Woman's Body
Women at Risk

This effort to value women is dedicated to:

my sister, Nela, who is a beautiful example of a Christian mother and teacher,

my mother-in-law, Lucille Carruth, and my mother, Ruth Hager, who have both gone on to their reward with the One who values women the most,

and four men who taught me how to honor and respect women—my father, Dr. C. R. Hager, who motivated me to write; Dr. Cecil Hamann and Dr. Paul Ray, who encouraged me to pursue a career in medicine; and Dr. John W. Greene, Jr., who taught me how important it is to care for the physical and emotional needs of women compassionately.

Contents

Preface

*e*ven though I was trained as a medical specialist in obstetrics and gynecology, it wasn't until I began to see how Jesus treated women that I understood how I, as a doctor, should treat them. I have also discovered that once women understand how Jesus treated and valued women, they come to value themselves as they ought.

In this book I want to pass along some of these discoveries to you. Basically, here is what I have found:

God values you as a woman and wants you to receive the same blessings and loving care Jesus demonstrated to women during His time on earth. I cannot emphasize enough how much He wants you to experience His forgiveness, compassion, mercy, and grace. God desires to inhabit you with His presence through His Holy Spirit and to enable you to experience the gifts of the Spirit: love, joy, peace, patience, kindness, goodness, gentleness, faithfulness, and self-control.

Jesus wants you to have total health—physical, emotional, and spiritual. As you read about His encounters with women in the Gospels, you will see that they had to first recognize their need, then reach out or be willing to be reached, have faith to believe that healing was possible, accept the healing in His time and way, and finally do what He told them to do afterward. From the hands of the Great Physician there is always something more, frequently requiring patience and trust. Jesus' healing touch gives total wholeness and peace, but not necessarily all at once, and perhaps not even on this side of eternity.

If you are suffering or are afraid, if you feel lonely and are without resources, please know that you are not alone. God is totally aware of your condition. He is moved with compassion and wants to meet your needs—the immediate always within the context of the eternal.

Jesus performed many miracles of healing, some of them instantaneously and some of them over time. Almost always, He included a spiritual admonition to change the person's way of life following the miracle. He knew that for real healing to take place, a change had to occur in the soul as well as in the body. This is why He regularly pronounced forgiveness of sins as He healed.

If you are looking to God for healing, seek Him for Himself more than for the healing. See Him as the Healer of your total self, of your desires, your decisions, your thoughts and actions, your frustrations and pains, your relational problems, your selfishness, and your dark side. Open yourself totally to God and know that He will probably ask you to make some changes in your way of life. Realize that what you are seeking right now from God may be only a part of what you need in order to become more like Him. Your request may fall short of what He desires for you to experience.

Because God created you, loves you, and knows your true needs, He also knows how you see yourself. As you ask Him for healing and change, ask Him also for a new vision of yourself and of your relationship with Him. Tell Him you want to see yourself as He sees you, and then be open to the One who offers you eternal life.

In these next chapters as we look at Jesus' interactions with women, I hope you will let Jesus meet you at your point of greatest need. He will surely be there for you, waiting with outstretched arms.

Acknowledgments

My gratitude goes out to Bill Petersen, a senior editor at Baker Book House, who responded to God's direction and encouraged me to write this book.

I'm also grateful to Carole Streeter, who persisted in drawing out of me the words to describe the way in which I attempt to minister as a physician to the physical, emotional, and spiritual needs of my patients.

Introduction

areful study of Jesus' life and ministry has challenged me to follow His example in my attitudes toward and treatment of women. But that hasn't been easy.

I should have had a very positive attitude toward women, because my father was a great example. He treated my mother with great respect and insisted that women should always be honored and never mistreated. I was reprimanded when I was mean to my sister or her friends, and talking back to my mother or showing even the slightest hint of disrespect was never allowed. I was instructed to say, "Yes, ma'am," and to open doors for women and girls. Never did I see a man strike a woman. Yet, in spite of this teaching and my father's example, my attitude toward women left much to be desired.

I remember one instance when I was only five or six years old and my mother and I were shopping for my school clothes. While Mom looked through a rack of pants, I wrestled with the arm of a mannequin to see if it was detachable. When the clerk noticed I was treating the model roughly, she asked me not to play with it and warned that it might fall on me. I immediately snapped back at her, "You can't tell me what to do!"

It took my mother less than three seconds to whisk me up and rush me into a nearby fitting room where she vigorously whacked me across the bottom. Then she did something all parents should do after punishing their children—she told me she loved me and explained why my behavior was inappropriate. "You must not be rude and unkind to other people," she told me. I tried to argue with her, but she continued, "You must show respect, even if you don't feel that a person deserves it."

As I grew older, I noticed how my parents always demonstrated respect for all people. As school superintendent, my father stood up against strong opposition to integrate the county school system. Members of a racial hate group confronted my mother at our front door one day while my father was gone, and she firmly but kindly refused to allow them to enter our home. I never heard disparaging racial or ethnic statements from my parents, and they never referred to women as being less able than men. My brother, sister, and I were instructed to treat others as we wished to be treated, regardless of sex or race.

Despite this teaching and my parents' example, however, I moved into adolescence without the attitudes and social skills necessary for respectful interaction with women. This was particularly evident in my dating relationships. I would date a girl for a while and then break off the relationship without explanation as soon as things began to get serious.

When I began dating Linda, who eventually became my wife, the same thing happened. But after breaking up and getting back together several times, our relationship did become more serious. One day, I told my father that I was planning to break up with Linda again. He sat me down and pointed to the root of the problem in all of these breakups. "David," he said, "you're afraid to commit to someone, and you don't show any respect in the way you treat the girls you date." He went on to say that God did not intend men to treat women with disrespect. His words deeply affected me, and I took the first step on a long and tortuous journey toward wholeness in my attitudes toward women. I continued dating Linda, and we have now been married nearly thirty years.

As my spiritual faith matured, I began to recognize the personal perceptions and biases that colored my views of people. God called me to strip away those biases and to see others as He sees them. Regardless of how they have treated me, I am called to respond to others with unconditional love. To care as I am cared for, to forgive as I am forgiven, to love as I am loved by the Father. My journey toward realizing this calling has prompted me to look to Jesus for my inspiration and to study the ways in which He interacted with women.

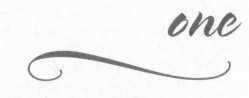

How Did Jesus Treat Women?

s you study the Bible, you will find that most men in biblical times did not have a high regard for women. They measured a woman's worth entirely in terms of her ability to serve them. In fact, a popular prayer in Jesus' time went something like this: "Lord, I thank Thee that I am neither a Gentile, a dog, nor a woman."

Jesus and the Status Quo

Unlike his contemporary male counterparts, Jesus always enhanced the position of women, though it meant going against the status quo. Jesus interacted with women primarily one-on-one, just as He deals with us today. Sometimes it was a moment of worship and praise as experienced by the woman at Simon's house (Mark 14:3–9), or a time of grief and anguish like that of the widow of Nain (Luke 7:11–15). There were occasions of gentle correction,

17

such as the time He forgave the woman caught in adultery (John 8:2–11), and instances of personal teaching like that He gave the woman at the well (John 4:5–42). Whatever their circumstances, Jesus met these women just as He meets us today, as individuals, face-to-face, eye-to-eye, heart-to-heart, and soul-to-soul.

Why did Jesus take these opportunities to give personal attention to and raise the level of women in His society?

- Jesus was not threatened by women. The security of His relationship to His Father and His confidence in His identity allowed Him to elevate women to the position they deserved without worrying about what society thought.
- Jesus recognized both the *animus* and *anima*—the male and female traits that exist within the human personality. He acknowledged the anima's need to express deep inner feelings and emotions, and He perceived the human need for understanding and soul nurture.
- Jesus realized that if He did not oppose the pervading opinions of the time and elevate women, it would never be done.

Jesus' actions toward women fit the framework of God's plan for His life. Mary affirmed that shortly after she received Gabriel's announcement that she would bear the Messiah. In the words of praise we call the Magnificat, she drew from Hannah's words and proclaimed Jesus' ministry to elevate the poor, the hungry, and the downtrodden. Surely women found their place in these categories. (See 1 Sam. 2:1–10 and Luke 1:46–55.)

Matthew's genealogy of Jesus also reveals God's desire to enhance the status of women. He includes four women, despite their tainted or questionable heritages:

- Tamar, a childless widow who was waiting to marry a brother of her dead husband, finally dressed as a prostitute to entice her father-in-law, Judah, and raise up progeny from his family (Genesis 38).
- Rahab, a woman of Jericho who was called a harlot or prostitute, concealed God's men at great personal risk (Josh. 2; 6:15–25).
- Ruth, a Moabitess whose ancestry should have prevented her from having a place with the people of Israel, saw her life course changed through Boaz, the Christ archetype. She became a grandmother to King David (Ruth 3–4).
- Bathsheba, who had committed adultery with King David, later bore Solomon to succeed him (2 Sam. 11:2–12:24).

With the inclusion of these women in Christ's ancestral tree, God identified with the sinner and the downtrodden. He lifted them to positions of honor and respect and used them to accomplish His purposes.

The four Gospels record Jesus doing the same. Because women were given a lower place in the society of Jesus' time, He intentionally sought to interact with them in a redemptive and restorative manner. He also demonstrated that women could be incorporated into ministry. As Jesus and His disciples traveled the countryside, they depended on the kindness of a group of women for financial support, encouragement, and practical help. Jesus chose to deliver some of His most important teachings to women—to Martha when her brother died (John 11:17–27), to the woman of Samaria (John 4:5–26), and to Mary Magdalene, the first to see Him after His resurrection (John 20:10–18).

Jesus taught us about worship as He received lavish anointing from the woman at Simon's home (Mark 14:6–9). He stood against society's double standard of gender discrimination in His interaction with a woman caught in adultery (John 8:2–11). He made a strong statement against racial and religious discrimination when He went out of His way to talk with the Samaritan woman beside the well and accepted her in spite of her background and behavior (John 4:7–26). The Phoenician woman begged Jesus to heal her daughter, and although He first seemed to reject her, He then extended both physical and spiritual healing (Matt. 15:21–28). He stood against the social stigma of the day when He accepted the woman with the issue of blood after she reached out to touch His garment, refusing to behave as though she had contaminated Him (Mark 5:25–34).

We must not forget that as Jesus reached out to women in His own day, He continues to reach out today with a willingness to overturn outmoded traditions and social taboos, to break through old prejudices, and to extend great honor to women. Jesus desires to elevate women and draw them into personal relationships with Himself. At the foot of the cross, the ground is level. There, the issue of equality finds its heart in our willingness to move in submission to the convicting power of the Holy Spirit.

That convicting power of the Holy Spirit has shown me that I cannot call myself a follower of Christ and still retain attitudes that are not consistent with His example. In my roles as husband, father, physician, and friend, it is essential that I value women and honor them for the strong, courageous, and special people they are.

The Modern Fight for Equality

Strong and impassioned movements spanning more than a century have seen women speaking up to establish their equality. As a result, their legal and occupational rights and roles have changed dramatically, so that women now have the right to vote, to hold public office, and to be ordained into ministry, and they are assuming expanding leadership roles and filling positions in the workplace on an equal status with men.

It seems strange to me, then, that so many women still hold the same negative attitudes about themselves as do some of the men in their lives. Yet I know that women learn much about who they are from their fathers and brothers, their boyfriends and husbands, their employers, and the men in their churches. When these men repeatedly treat women in a condescending or cruel manner and frequently regard them as servants or second-class citizens, women subconsciously come to believe the message that they are somehow inferior. One part of them knows it is not true, but when women constantly encounter put-downs, exclusion, and male prejudices, they often find it easier to acquiesce than to fight.

Many Christian women experience demeaning attitudes even in their own churches. Seldom, if ever, do they hear about how Jesus reached through walls of paternalistic tradition and prejudice to elevate women and assure them of His love and support. Although there are honest differences of belief about the place of women in the church, even the most restrictive Christian churches should encourage men to demonstrate the Spirit of Christ in the honor they give to women.

Barriers to Self-Esteem

Among the women I have interviewed, the two most common barriers to positive self-esteem are lack of communication and self-neglect. Two places where women should be confident of open communication are the home and the church. Yet I often hear from my patients that their pleas to be heard fall on deaf ears in both places. I would like to excuse the problem with a plea that men are not good listeners, but I know that often we simply refuse to hear what the women near us say. As little boys in men's bodies, "girl talk" frightens us and makes us feel insecure. I am sure I am not the only man who feels comfortable speaking to large groups but has had trouble learning how to communicate on an intimate level with his wife.

Self-neglect, the second barrier to positive self-esteem, is something I have seen in many of my patients. In their conscientiousness and sense of obligation toward others, they take better care of their children and husbands, their friends, their homes and offices, their cars, and even their pets, than they do of themselves, seriously minimizing the importance of their own well-being. Over time, this lack of self-care makes physical and spiritual health deteriorate.

What constitutes healthy self-care? The culture of the '90s is full of convoluted and conflicting messages. Extreme feminism, New Age spiritualism, and societal immorality scream from all directions, leading to an identity conflict and recurrent questions. "Should I follow career or personhood or marriage?" "Should I be strong or coy?" "Should I work outside the home?" "Can I be satisfied in life as a single person?" Because their pace of life is so hectic, many women never pause long enough to make careful decisions about these matters. Only a loving heavenly Father can lead them through the frantic mazes and into a place of peace and grace. It is difficult to hear His voice, however, when they are burdened by excessive demands of work, family, and friends. It takes time to listen to God, but these times of meditation are important because this is when God can impress upon the listener that her true worth and value is found in the intimacy of her relationship with Him.

A Doctor's Prescription for Better Health

If you sometimes wonder about your place in God's plan, are tired of being tired, and feel that the candle you are burning at both ends is slowly burning out, remember that God has made you in His image. Psalm 139 says that He wove you together in your mother's womb, where you were fearfully and wonderfully made. God did the weaving and making of you, He knows the substance of which you are made, and He has ordained the days of your life. Because of this, He has more respect for your strengths, hope for your potential, patience with your failings, and tenderness toward your hurts than you do. So you can truly say with the psalmist,

> Search me, O God, and know my heart;
> test me and know my anxious thoughts.
> See if there is any offensive way in me,
> and lead me in the way everlasting.
> Psalm 139:23–24

When you are confused, God wants to lead you. When you feel trapped in a pit so deep you don't think anyone can hear you, much less pull you out, He wants to liberate you. When you are hurting, He wants to heal you. When you have failed and need forgiveness, He reaches to you with grace and pardon. When you are exhausted or confused, He wants to give you rest. Jesus said, "Come to me, all you who are weary and burdened, and I will give you rest" (Matt. 11:28). The Hebrew idea of *rest* and the sabbath instituted for such rest was "to hide away." The Lord wants to hide you away in a rest that only He can provide. That doesn't mean that you will have no more work, but rather that He will hold you and comfort you when you are tired and ready to give up. He will refresh and renew you.

It is important for you to respect your own needs and desires. One part of you has an innate compulsion to give and give. But if you spend all of your time and energy meeting the needs and desires of your children or your spouse or your friends at the expense of your own well-being, you will eventually feel overlooked and rejected. Then you will become angry—at first mildly so, but eventually very angry. When you add that anger to any pre-existing disease or condition, major health problems and ongoing emotional distress result.

How should you react to such situations? First, realize that you have resources available to you for dealing with the problem. This means, however, that you need to spend some time thinking and praying about your life—about your needs and your dreams, about your commitments and your desires.

You also need to think deeply about the fact that you are made in the image of God, who wants to draw you into close fellowship with Himself. Begin by accepting Jesus Christ as your personal Savior and then engage the ongoing process of coming to maturity in your faith and understanding of the Christian journey. Rely on God for your daily needs, not just for crisis provision. Spend time studying the Bible, receiving what the Holy Spirit wants to say to you individually. Set aside regular times for prayer as you praise, intercede, or petition God. Finally, surround yourself with friends who can hold you accountable and help you along your journey, even as you help them.

two

Please Help
My Child

*t*he biting chill of the wind cut through my sports
coat, and I shivered. Although it was unusually
cold for December in Kentucky, I welcomed the
fresh air. After two days on call at the hospital, I wondered
how I would manage to stay awake during a full day of
patient visits.

As I entered the office and donned my white coat, I saw
a note to call Marsha Smith as soon as possible. She had
been my patient for over ten years, and I assumed her call
was to request a prescription refill. But when I returned
Marsha's call, I found out her concern was for her daughter. She asked if Carrie could come for counseling as well
as a physical examination, but first Marsha wanted to
come in to talk with me alone, without Carrie.

Marsha told me that Carrie was a vivacious and attractive sixteen-year-old—the apple of her father's eye. She
was also an excellent student, an accomplished pianist,
and a fine gymnast. That is, she was all of these things
until a few months ago, when she suddenly began stay-

ing away from home, neglecting her piano practice and gymnastic training, and avoiding her church youth group. Instead of her former sweetness and positive attitude, she was now angry, resentful, and secretive.

Marsha acknowledged that she might be part of the problem. "I wanted so much for her to be a Christian and to grow up in an environment of love and forgiveness that I forced her to go to church and Bible study. In my over-zealousness and excessive protection, I allowed no room for her to be an individual. I know I did a lot of shaming and blaming, and now she is rebelling against me and against God."

Marsha paused before continuing, "I'm sure that our marital difficulties have added to the problem. I put a lot of pressure on Greg to be a success at work, to spend time with the family, and to be involved in church activities."

I recalled that at first Marsha and Greg's problems had seemed to be about religion. After becoming a Christian, Marsha devoted most of her time to church activities. This created a barrier between her and Greg, since he didn't want anything to do with the church. Marsha also had a problem controlling her personal spending, and the resulting financial strain added to the difficulties at home. Greg often reminded Marsha that her Christianity had made no difference in the way she lived her life on a daily basis. Yet he wasn't attempting to alter his dysfunctions either.

The couple separated for a while but had recently tried to reconcile. Marsha had entered counseling, hoping to resolve their marital differences, but Greg refused to go to the sessions, claiming he had no problems that needed resolution.

The more Marsha and Greg talked, the worse things got in their marriage. Marsha is a woman of prayer, and she surrounded herself with friends who joined her in peti-tioning God on behalf of the marriage and for Greg's sal-vation. It was during this period of intense prayer that Greg became more and more angry, finally resulting in violent verbal abuse. This turned into physical abuse when Marsha refused to give up her participation in her prayer group or church activities. After the counselor advised another separation, Marsha left Greg but did not pursue divorce.

Marsha was in the deepest quagmire of her life. She had seen her marriage come to a traumatic separation, and now her daughter was threatening to reject her. As she tried to go on, she began to sob hysterically. "I don't know what to do, Dr. Hager."

"Marsha, you are going to make it," I said. "You need to believe that."

Later that week when I met Carrie, my first impression was that she was lonely, bitter, and very angry. I knew this would be a tough session.

"Carrie, tell me something about yourself."

"What do you want to know?" she responded, without raising her head to look at me.

"Just tell me about things you like to do, places you go, and . . ."

"What did my mother tell you about the places I go?"

"She didn't tell me anything about them. I just want to hear about you."

For several minutes Carrie was quiet. Finally, I said, "Look, we both have other things we need to do, so why don't you go ahead and leave. I'll be here whenever you are ready to talk."

Two weeks later, Carrie called the office wanting to speak with me. She didn't apologize for her previous silence but asked if I would talk with her the next day. I thought about putting her off for a few days, to see if she were serious, but then decided this might be my only chance to talk with her. We agreed on 5:00 the next afternoon.

When she entered my office, Carrie was still sad and withdrawn, but at least she was willing to talk. "I just don't understand why she is so worried about me. If she would spend more time taking care of herself, maybe she would still be with my father."

"Carrie, I know that you love your father very much, and you want your parents to get back together again. I believe they will, but for now, it may be best if they have some time to work out their individual problems. I think you also need to work on your issues so that when the family is reunited it will be stronger."

Once Carrie began talking, I didn't need to ask any questions. "Mom and Dad always fought. I know she had to make him leave because he was hitting her, but where does this leave me with Dad? I miss him a lot more than you know. When he left, he was leaving me too." She paused and then went on, "I could never meet their expectations. My grades weren't good enough. I never performed as well as Dad thought I should in gymnastics, and I'll never play the piano as well as Mom does. I just don't measure up to their standards.

"Mom made me go to church, and I totally hated it. The youth minister was always telling us that we were terrible people who were all going straight to hell. I'm like, 'Isn't God supposed to be this loving father type? Could we possibly hear something about that?'

"It was totally the pits! None of my friends did church, and so I started spending Saturday nights with them so I wouldn't have to go on Sunday. They partied a lot, and we always had a great time."

"Carrie, was there drinking and drugs at these parties?"

"Well, sure," she responded. "There's drinking and stuff at all parties. You have kids—don't you know that? I started smoking cigarettes and drinking beer; if I hadn't, the other kids wouldn't have hung out with me."

Carrie said that beer gave way to hard liquor and cigarettes to pot. Soon she began dating a guy who had dropped out of high school. Her friends encouraged her to come to special parties held in a field outside of town.

There everyone got high; then they built a big bonfire and threw live animals into the flames. This was followed by satanic worship during which the guys took turns having sex with all the girls.

"Mom found my birth control pills in my room one night and went ballistic. I left home and stayed with a friend for two weeks. When I needed money to pay for drugs, I called Dad. He always gave me what I wanted so he wouldn't feel guilty about not being at home.

"I didn't feel right about the cult or about my friends, but they accepted me the way I was. I can't give up my drugs or my type of worship. It makes me feel good about myself. I know you don't understand—you probably think just like my mother."

When Carrie left the office, I had a strong feeling that this was not our last meeting.

A Phoenician Daughter in Need

Marsha and Carrie's situation reminds me of a story about Jesus and another mother and daughter. Both Matthew (15:21–28) and Mark (7:24–30) tell about a woman from Phoenicia whom Jesus encountered when He and His disciples traveled to the cities of Tyre and Sidon, where the people worshiped the god Baal and the goddess Astarte.

Jesus was evidently seeking rest from His constant pace of teaching and healing. Mark says, "He entered a house and did not want anyone to know it; yet he could not keep his presence secret" (7:24). Most of us know this feeling. Even though I love my work, there are times when the demands of people nearly suck the life out of me, and I have to escape in solitude. Sometimes getting away means a vacation or weekend in a place where no one can reach me by phone and perhaps no one knows me. Occasionally I have to take a personal retreat to pray, meditate, and allow my battery to be recharged.

This must have been such a time for Jesus. Yet, His reputation preceded Him. As soon as He arrived, He was besieged by a desperate mother.

This woman must have wondered whether she would be accepted—she was a Greek entering a Jewish home to appeal to a Hebrew prophet. What if the owner of the house forced her to leave? Most Jewish men would not bother themselves with the concerns of a Jewish woman. How could she expect any sympathy when she was not of His faith? Yet this mother showed unusual boldness in approaching Jesus without introduction and falling at His feet to plead for her daughter. And when Jesus didn't respond to her in a positive way, she demonstrated the depth of her faith in a unique exchange.

The Phoenician mother told Jesus that her daughter was possessed by a demon or unclean spirit. This may have been actual demon possession, or it could have indicated that she was mentally unstable, was prone to seizures, or had a behavior disorder. We do know that the girl's actions had become so unpleasant or dangerous that her mother was willing to beg for help.

Today we might say that demonic possession is a result of persistent sin or experimentation with the occult so that Satan is allowed to exert his control in the person's life. Or in some cases the evil spirit may be present as a result of generational sin. Just as Marsha felt guilty about her role in Carrie's problems, so this Phoenician mother may have felt she was somehow responsible for her daughter's difficulties.

Many mothers come to a time when they are so desperate to find help for a child that their own pride no longer matters; all they want is mercy for the son or daughter they love. When these mothers come to God to ask for help, they expect a better reception than the Phoenician woman received. Matthew tells us Jesus didn't even answer her (15:23). When she continued her persistent crying out, the disciples urged Jesus to send her away. He said to them, "I was sent only to the lost sheep of Israel" (15:24). Was this statement a test to the disciples or a reminder of their primary mission? We don't know.

The Phoenician mother was persistent. She was not about to be brushed off, for she pushed her way through the disciples to kneel before Jesus, imploring, "Lord, help me!" (Matt. 15:25). Now, we think, Jesus will show her kindness. But to our surprise, He said, "First let the children eat all they want, . . . for it is not right to take the children's bread and toss it to their dogs" (Mark 7:27). By this He meant that it would not be right for Him to bestow a blessing intended for the Jews on someone who was less than a child of promise.

It is hard to believe Jesus would answer her in such an insensitive way. Yet there must have been something in His tone or the look on His face that encouraged her to retort, "Yes, Lord, . . . but even the dogs under the table eat the children's crumbs" (Mark 7:28). She acknowledged that as a Gentile she was willing to take the leavings from the table of the Jews, but as a mother she was not giving up until Jesus healed her daughter. He was overwhelmed by her persistence and faith, and He told her that she could return home where she would find her daughter healed.

How would you or I respond if confronted by rejection when our child's health was at stake? Would we fly into a frenzy, threaten physical violence, or determinedly try to find help elsewhere? When our children are suffering, we will go to great extremes to see that their needs are met. When they hurt, we hurt—sitting up at night with a sick child, rushing to calm the fears of a bad dream, or treating cuts and scrapes with kisses and bandages are all nat-

ural expressions of our love and dedication. When we feel
they have been falsely accused or unfairly treated, we rise
to their defense. When they have a chronic disease, we
rearrange our lives to meet their needs. At other times,
when tough love is necessary, our child's pain is still our
pain because it is not easy to allow our children to experience the grievous consequences of their behavior. But no
matter what the situation, the best thing we can do for
our children is to take the problem to God in prayer. There
is no greater gift that parents can give their children. I will
never forget the many times I saw my mother on her knees
praying for me and my safety when I tried to sneak into
the house late at night after breaking curfew. Her devotion and persistence in prayer made an indelible mark on
my life.

The Case of a Misguided Mother

Peggy was another mother who sought help for her
child, but she was far off the mark as she diagnosed her
teenage daughter's problem. Peggy brought Candy to my
office during a school break a few years ago because she
was concerned that her daughter was no longer having
periods. Candy had begun menstruating when she was
twelve, but after two years of normal menstruation, she
had not even spotted for the past two years. Peggy was
afraid her daughter had some type of tumor.

As the three of us sat in my office, I observed that Candy
was unusually thin and apparently very shy. Her mother
answered all the questions for the medical history. What
astonished me was that she never mentioned anything
about Candy's weight; she was seemingly oblivious to the
fact that her daughter was practically skin and bones. As
I asked more questions intended for Candy, Peggy contin-

ued to answer, and I realized that I was getting nowhere fast. So I suggested that I examine Candy in order to see if there were physical problems. I insisted that Peggy wait in my office—I wanted a chance to talk directly with Candy.

When we were in the examining room, I could tell that Candy was frightened, and so I asked her questions about school, her voice lessons, dance class, and her church youth group. She was a very busy young lady who had little time for herself; she appeared to be under a great deal of stress. As we continued to talk, it became obvious that the major source of stress in her life was her mother. Peggy had pressured her daughter into all of her activities and made it clear that mere involvement was not enough; she had to excel.

Candy felt pressured by her coach as well as her mother to keep her weight down. Peggy frequently told Candy that she was getting fat and wouldn't be able to make a good impression or compete in public dance and voice competition. As a result, Candy would begin to diet whenever she went over one hundred pounds, even though she was five feet five inches tall. Purging, by inducing vomiting and diarrhea, kept her weight at eighty-five to eighty-eight pounds.

When I told Peggy privately that I thought Candy was anorectic, she was flabbergasted. She denied the possibility and insisted that I was mistaken, but the signs and symptoms were obvious.

Anorexia nervosa affects approximately 1 percent of adolescent and young adult women. In my practice, I am seeing an increasing number of young women with this disorder. Unfortunately, it is very difficult to manage, and the mortality rate is as high as 20 percent. This is usually the result of starvation and its related metabolic effects and sometimes from suicide.[1]

As we talked about the pressure Candy felt to succeed, Peggy began to cry. After she composed herself, she said,

"I was anorectic when I was Candy's age. I was never able to succeed at the things Candy is good at, and I just want her to have some of the happiness I never knew."

"Peggy, the best way for you and your husband to make your daughter happy is to let her know that she doesn't have to perform in order to have your love. Let her know that you want her to be well, not so that she can perform but so that she can feel better. How would you respond if she gave up voice and dance lessons? Has she been able to be a little girl, an adolescent? She just wants you to love her for who she is, not for what she does." I then asked if I could pray for them, and I brought Candy back into the room.

I would like to tell you that this family had no more problems, but that is not the case. However, they are in counseling and are on the road to recovery. They are learning to love each other for who they are.

The Healing Process

As we look at the biblical story of the Phoenician woman and her daughter and then at more modern stories of mothers and children, I want to remind you of some principles about healing:

- Illness involves the physical, emotional, and spiritual aspects of our lives. Sickness in one area touches all the others.
- Healing, then, must also touch the total person—the physical, emotional, and spiritual.
- When we ask for healing, we need to trust God's timing. Healing may be immediate, gradual, delayed, or eternal.
- For healing to take place, someone must see and express the need, whether it be physical, emotional,

spiritual, or a combination. God's desire is that we be whole, but He wants us to acknowledge at least to some degree what we need.

- Although love and devotion are usually behind the pursuit of health for a family member, they are not enough in themselves. Faith must also be present for healing to occur.
- If we do not see immediate results, we should not be discouraged from continuing in prayer as well as seeking appropriate medical help.
- There needs to be a recognition of sin and unworthiness, a condition we all share. Many of Jesus' healing miracles combined physical restoration with forgiveness of sins.
- When we see evidence that healing has occurred, we should give thanks and praise to the Great Physician.

Even with divine intervention, the healing process may take a long time. At the beginning of this chapter, I began the story of Marsha and Carrie. Following those events, I scheduled a conference with Marsha to discuss these principles of healing. I was also concerned about the emotions Marsha must be feeling and asked whether she was dealing with anger, bitterness, resentment, or jealousy.

As we talked, I suggested that Marsha needed to evaluate her relationship with God and her husband before she could expect to successfully intercede with the Great Physician. Then I asked her to read some verses from the Bible about winning her husband to the Lord:

> Wives, fit in with your husbands' plans; for then if they refuse to listen when you talk to them about the Lord, they will be won by your respectful, pure behavior. Your godly lives will speak to them better than any words.

Don't be concerned about the outward beauty that
depends on jewelry, or beautiful clothes, or hair arrange-
ments. Be beautiful inside, in your hearts, with the lasting
charm of a gentle and quiet spirit which is so precious to
God. That kind of deep beauty was seen in the saintly
women of old, who trusted God and fitted in with their husbands' plans.

1 Peter 3:1–5 (TLB)

It was important for Marsha to examine her relationship with God, because she was the one who would need
to have faith that the evil spirit in Carrie would be exor-
cised. Just as the Phoenician woman pled with Jesus to
heal her daughter, Marsha would intercede that her beautiful child, full of God's presence, would be restored to her.

Carrie was not immediately healed, but Marsha continued in faithful persistence and prayer. Some months
later I received a letter from Carrie from a rehabilitation
center where she was undergoing treatment for narcotic
addiction. She said she had changed her circle of friends
and was losing her desire for tobacco and alcohol. Also,
she had terminated sexual intimacy with her boyfriend
and would be living at home again when the treatment
was finished. She had not returned to church, and she was
still angry at her father, but I believe these matters will be
resolved as well—in time. God heard the cry of a desperate mother, and the healing process has begun.

Parenting 101

Marsha took a step that many parents do not—she
sought help. Many parents think they can resolve the
problems their children face on their own, or they feel
revealing the issue will cause embarrassment, it will
demean them and reflect on their abilities as parents, or

others will think they don't have the resources to keep their homes in order. Yet, if we are honest, we all know that we require help and advice in dealing with our families.

Parenting 101 isn't offered when we have babies. We all learn by experience and by accepting wise counsel from others and applying it to our own situation so that we can guide our children in the best way possible. Even with a healthy childrearing plan, we must individualize those concepts to meet the needs of each child's unique personality, desires, and motivations. We can hold to basic concepts, but we need to be flexible in ensuring that each child perceives his or her own self-worth and recognizes that he or she is a unique creation of God, loved for who he or she is by the heavenly Father as well as earthly parents.

three

Infertility, Adoption, and Miracle Babies

One of the most exciting events in life is the birth of a child. I also believe that it is one of the most blessed and sacred events in life. In His wisdom, God designed the mystical experience of sexual intimacy to unite a couple in love and to provide for the propagation of the race. Because He made this intimate relationship, we know that God takes great joy in the birth of each child—even those born into homes where life will not be as nurturing as it should be.

Unfortunately, not everyone is able to experience the miracle of conception and birth. For some people this is because of life choices; for others it is a result of physical factors.

A Child in Her Old Age

Zechariah and his wife, Elizabeth, were direct descendants from the levitical line of Aaron, the brother of Moses who became the first high priest of Israel. Zechariah and Elizabeth were "well along in years" but had no children because Elizabeth was barren or infertile (Luke 1:7). In biblical times, barrenness was the greatest curse a Jewish woman could endure. Not only were there no children to help with the family labors, but there would be no heir to carry on the family name. Their childlessness was a grief to this couple.

Then an angel of the Lord came to Zechariah as he was serving in the temple and told him that his aged wife would yet bear him a son who would "go on before the Lord, in the spirit and power of Elijah . . . to make ready a people prepared for the Lord" (Luke 1:17). Unable to believe such a thing, Zechariah asked for a sign that this would really occur. The angel Gabriel told him that because of his doubt he would be unable to speak until Elizabeth gave birth (v. 20). When he finished his priestly service, Zechariah left the temple in a state of dazed but silent joy.

I can relate to Zechariah. I tend to be very realistic, and when the numbers do not add up, I generally believe they never will. Because of this, I have had to learn to accept that God can do anything, no matter how improbable the odds. My wife, Linda, on the other hand, is very perceptive and can believe that God can and will do whatever He says. She has an innate level of trust far greater than mine. If she and I had been in the places of Zechariah and Elizabeth, I think God would have struck me speechless, while Linda would have been out telling our friends about the great miracle God was about to do.

Unlike her husband, Elizabeth embraced the angel's unbelievable message without doubt and praised God for taking away her curse. "'The Lord has done this for me,' she said. 'In these days he has shown his favor and taken away my disgrace among the people'" (Luke 1:25).

Elizabeth's response was very much like Mary's, when Gabriel announced to her that she would conceive and bear the Messiah. The women asked for no sign but simply submitted to the will of their heavenly Father with joy and faith.

Mary traveled to the hill country outside Jerusalem to visit with her cousin Elizabeth, and when Elizabeth saw Mary, she was filled with the Holy Spirit and exclaimed:

> Blessed are you among women, and blessed is the child you will bear! But why am I so favored, that the mother of my Lord should come to me? As soon as the sound of your greeting reached my ears, the baby in my womb leaped for joy. Blessed is she who has believed that what the Lord has said to her will be accomplished!
>
> Luke 1:42–45

In an aging, infertile wife and in an innocent, adolescent virgin, God found faithful and obedient women who would bear the special children of His purpose. A person's age, position, or experience is not the deciding factor. God is looking for people of faith who will trust Him in every part of life. Through the children born to Mary and Elizabeth, God would reveal His plan of salvation for all people.

Mary remained with Elizabeth, sharing the miracles God was performing in their lives, until shortly before Elizabeth gave birth to the son whom Gabriel had said should be named John. As Zechariah wrote the name of his son for those who had gathered to rejoice with them, he regained his speech. Baby John would one day be called John the Baptist, and as Gabriel foretold, he was filled with the Holy Spirit and prepared the way for the Messiah, who was born to Mary just a few months later.

Miraculous Births

Senior citizens don't produce babies, and that is exactly why the story of Zechariah and Elizabeth is so miraculous.

Nor do couples considered infertile for thirteen years usually conceive, especially when they have decided against further medical help. But God answered the prayers of Catherine and Don and gave them the desire of their hearts.

All through the Bible, we read of God's involvement with the conception and birth of particular babies. He is deeply interested in the fertility and reproductive potential of His children. We read in Psalm 139:13–16:

> For you created my inmost being;
>   you knit me together in my mother's womb.
> I praise you because I am fearfully and wonderfully made;
>   your works are wonderful,
>   I know that full well.
> My frame was not hidden from you
>   when I was made in the secret place.
> When I was woven together in the depths of the earth,
>   your eyes saw my unformed body.

The Lord told the prophet Jeremiah, "Before I formed you in the womb I knew you, before you were born I set you apart" (Jer. 1:5).

Just as God is involved in our creation, so He is interested in conception:

- God informed Abraham that Sarah would become pregnant with Isaac when she was ninety years old (Gen. 17:15–21).
- In the time of the judges, an angel came to Manoah and his wife to tell them that although she was sterile, she would bear a son who would "begin the deliverance of Israel from the hands of the Philistines" (Judg. 13:5). The child born to them was Samson, the strongest man in the world.
- The angel Gabriel announced the birth of John to Zechariah and then told Mary that she was blessed

among women and would conceive God's own son,
Jesus (Luke 1:11–20, 26–38).

Remarkable miracles of conception still occur. Catherine was thirty-seven years old when she first came to see me. She and Don were both only children, and they were under extreme pressure to produce some offspring. Don in particular had a great desire for his family name to continue. But they had been trying unsuccessfully to conceive for thirteen years. They had never sought medical care for this problem and had virtually given up all hope of having children.

Aging is one of the leading causes of infertility—after the age of thirty-five, success in conceiving becomes increasingly more difficult for most women. The number of eggs in a woman's ovaries is determined at conception. At the time of an infant girl's birth, the number of eggs is approximately a million. By the first menstrual period, the number is under 400,000. This number slowly decreases over a woman's reproductive years, and by age thirty-five the number of viable eggs is drastically reduced. Because the remaining eggs are fewer, conception is less likely to occur, and because they are older, they are also more likely to have genetic alterations.

Catherine and Don knew that their chances of conceiving were remote. We initiated a workup including blood tests, documentation of ovulation, an X ray to determine if Catherine's fallopian tubes were open, and a semen analysis to see if Don's sperm count was normal.[1] The test results indicated that Catherine was not ovulating regularly and Don had an abnormality in his sperm motility.

We took steps to assist reproduction by stimulating regular ovulation with medication, enhancing the motility of Don's sperm, and then inoculating his sperm into Catherine's uterus. After six unsuccessful cycles, they decided they did not have the emotional energy, patience, or money to pursue any further attempts to conceive. I accepted their decision, prayed with them, and told them that I would pray for them regularly regarding a pregnancy. Don seemed to dismiss the idea, but Catherine remained hopeful.

Three months after her thirty-eighth birthday, Catherine called to tell me of a dream in which she was told that she would conceive. She was convinced that God had spoken to her in this dream and that she would have a baby. She had waited to call me until she was a week late on her period. We ran a blood pregnancy test, and to our surprise and delight, it was positive! Needless to say, Catherine and Don were ecstatic and humbled that God had heard the petitions of their hearts and had granted them what our medical attempts had failed to produce.

Catherine had a difficult pregnancy, but she carried to term and delivered a beautiful baby girl. This precious little one is her parents' pride and joy. Although they have not conceived again, Catherine and Don are praising the Creator for the gift of their little girl.

Facing Unfulfilled Dreams

We know that many fertility problems do not end in a successful pregnancy. If you have not been able to conceive, you have probably talked with many friends and physicians about your fertility problem. (By the way, I always use the phrase "fertility problem" rather than "infertility problem" because it is more positive.) I understand the frustration of going through test after test, procedure after procedure without having a child. This stirs up feelings of anger or guilt, which may have no obvious explanation or which may be directed at the spouse whose physical problem or past actions cause the infertility.

Sometimes infertility is the result of choices people make. Some who were sexually active in earlier years contracted diseases that affected the genital tract. Pelvic inflammatory disease is a sexually transmitted infection that can completely or partially block the fallopian tubes. A sexually transmitted virus, human papilloma virus, causes over 90 percent of all precancerous and cancerous disease of the cervix. When it is treated, there is the possibility that the cervix can be narrowed so that sperm cannot pass freely. Other diseases such as endometriosis, thyroid disease, and chronic problems such as renal disease and lupus can affect fertility. In spite of everything that reproductive endocrinologists can do, conception may not occur.

Increasingly today we see couples who have delayed a family in favor of two careers and financial security. Many young people want to complete their education, get established in a good job, purchase a home, and be financially stable before they even think of having children. When both spouses work outside the home, the pressures and demands of their vocations often leave them tired and stressed to the point that being sexually intimate, much less having a child, is remote from their minds. Unfortunately, as with Catherine and Don, age can be a major factor in fertility, and while I am not suggesting that couples should have children before they are ready, they should be aware that a long delay may affect their reproductive potential.

Sometimes a physical obstruction affects a successful pregnancy. This was the case with Alice and Brad. They came to see me after two first-trimester pregnancy losses. They had been cared for by another physician and, as so frequently happens after a pregnancy loss, did not feel comfortable returning to their former doctor because of the painful memories.

Alice conceived again before a pregnancy-loss workup could be initiated, and she miscarried for the third time.

She missed her follow-up appointment, and three months later the same thing happened again. Finally, we were able to evaluate Alice and found that she had a septum (a membranous division) inside the uterus that decreased the area available for normal placental development and caused her to miscarry. When we surgically removed the septum via a hysteroscope,[2] she conceived and carried the baby to term.

Alice and Brad were thrilled with their baby girl, but they also remembered their days of grief. They are now involved with the pregnancy-loss program at a local hospital and continue to comfort grieving couples, some of whom may never have a live-born infant.

If you have been unable to have biological children, have tried every avenue available, and feel heartbroken, I want to assure you that God sees and feels your pain. Even if you are so angry and bitter that you can't believe He cares, God wants to comfort you in your grief and frustration through His Holy Spirit and often through the loving care of other Christians.

Adoption Love

Whatever your situation, do not allow your pain, anger, or bitterness to control your life to the extent that you are perpetually sad. I have seen childless women who allow their lack of fertility to rob them of every other opportunity for joy. They seem to wear a scowl all the time, and this really affects the quality of their marriages.

Many others, however, are open to considering the option of adoption. When I mention this to a childless couple, their first response is usually, "We just want our own child. We don't think we could raise someone else's."

It is normal to prefer to have our own biological offspring. But another way to look at adoption is to remember that God is the Creator of all life, and all children—adopted or biological—are truly His children. I believe that some people have been specially chosen by God to become parents to one or more children who otherwise would not have caring parents.

Kathy and Rob had gone through extensive evaluation for fertility, and yet we could find no cause for their childlessness. They had been through laparoscopy,[3] artificial insemination with Rob's sperm, and in-vitro fertilization procedures. Finally, I suggested that they consider adoption. Their response was just as I expected: "We are not cut out to raise somebody else's baby." I suggested that they think about it for a while. Three months later they called to ask if I would put them on our adoption list. I was glad to do this but also advised them to contact all of the adoption agencies as well as other obstetricians. They then went through the state-legislated process of being approved as adoptive parents.

About a year later, Kathy called our office to tell us that they were going to become parents of a beautiful baby from South America. How thrilled they were to bring little Samuel in to see us. When Samuel was a year old, they were asked if they wanted to adopt an American biracial child, and they readily accepted.

As they were getting ready to pick up the baby in another state, Kathy began to experience severe nausea and vomiting. She was evaluated by her family physician, even having an endoscopic procedure to rule out an ulcer. When she called me about her symptoms, I asked when her last period had been. She said, "I really don't know. We've been so busy with the adoption work and making plans to leave." She laughed when I suggested she come by the office for a pregnancy test. "Dr. Hager, there is no way that I could be pregnant. We tried for over ten years and never conceived once."

You can imagine how pleased we all were when the pregnancy test was positive. Kathy and Rob now have three beautiful children. They were obedient to God's call to adopt two of His little children who might not have survived in their original surroundings, and then they were blessed with a biological child.

Besides bringing joy to the lives of infertile couples, adoption also provides a positive alternative to the tragedy of abortion. Presently, 42 percent of unmarried teens who conceive decide to abort them. I would like to see these teens choosing instead to give birth to their babies and to place them for adoption if they decide not to keep them. While the problem of unwanted pregnancy is complex, one of the solutions is to encourage those who do not want to raise the child to give birth and allow their precious ones to be adopted by people like Kathy and Rob.

Medical Intervention

As a Christian physician, I am frequently asked to give my opinion on assisted reproduction. Should any means other than intercourse between husband and wife be used to aid fertility? Is it right to inseminate an egg outside the body and reintroduce it into the mother? Is it right to use donor sperm or donor eggs? What about surrogate parenting?

Ideally, all married couples would be able to conceive on their own, but unfortunately, that just doesn't occur. Fifteen percent of couples in this country are infertile. Others are able to conceive but never have a live-born infant. This means that great numbers of couples seek care as fertility patients. I don't pretend to know all the answers to these sensitive matters, but after praying and seeking God's direction, I have come to some guidelines that I follow.

I believe God has given us intelligence and inquisitiveness that enable us to discover many things that medically enhance and prolong our lives. It is possible for people to use these advances well or to misuse them. Just as fire can cook food and provide light but also injure and destroy, so the field of medicine can also help or harm. We have medications that can stimulate a woman to ovulate, and some of these medications increase the chance of multiple births. We also have techniques such as intrauterine insemination and in-vitro fertilization that enable couples to conceive when they would otherwise be unable to do so.[4] I believe such techniques are wonderful medical advances.

The ethical questions arise when these procedures are performed on anyone other than a married couple. Should a woman other than the man's wife be impregnated with his sperm and carry the baby for the couple? I personally do not believe that surrogate parenting is ethically right. I also believe that the use of donor eggs or sperm to achieve a pregnancy raises many legal, emotional, and moral problems. I have seen marriages end soon after the birth of a child whose biological father was not the husband of the baby's mother. Each person, each couple, must take these matters to God and seek His direction after consulting His Word and listening to the counsel of godly pastors and trusted friends.

Answered Prayer

Some people don't think of childlessness as an illness that requires healing, and yet it causes deep pain for many couples and their families. Some couples desire to have children so much that they are willing to push to any lengths of medical intervention to conceive. In doing so, however, they may be interfering with God's plan and protection for their lives.

One of my patients experienced seven miscarriages (most while using medical intervention) before conceiving a baby with multiple congenital anomalies. It is possible, although still difficult, to imagine that this woman's difficulty in having a biological child might have been a form of protection that medical intervention neutralized.

Given the intense anguish and heartache of those couples who so strongly desire to have biological children but physically struggle to do so, it is very appropriate to pray that God will work in the lives of such couples. He designed our miraculous bodies, and He knows how to fix anything that is wrong or lacking in them. It is imperative, then, to call on Him to heal the physical and emotional scars of childlessness as He sees fit.

God cares about every circumstance surrounding birth and the desire to have children. He wants us to come to Him with all our cares and concerns, believing that He will answer in His way and His time. For some people, God's plan seems to be that they remain single or childless, possibly protecting them from unforeseeable heartaches. Although we cannot see God's plan or understand all of His guidance, we can trust ourselves to His loving protection and provision, believing that in *all* things a Father who is perfect in wisdom, love, and power is able to work good for those who love Him and are called according to His deep purposes (see Rom. 8:28).

Marianne's Prayer

When our children grow up and marry, we tend to assume grandchildren will eventually follow. At least that's what Marianne thought. Her daughter had already made her a proud grandma twice, and now the whole family was looking forward to the time when her son and his wife would have a baby. After Luke and Karen had been married several years, Marianne found out that they were beginning to seek help from a fertility specialist. This came as quite a shock to her—she had just taken for granted that nature would take its course, and it hadn't.

Marianne's church held small prayer services for healing, and one week she went to the chapel with the special intention of praying for Luke and Karen. As she knelt at the altar rail and the pastor came to her, Marianne could hardly get the words out to tell him that her prayer was for her son and his wife to have a child. She was anointed and prayed for, in the confidence that God would hear her loving request for her children.

Luke and Karen continued with their doctor and still nothing happened, except a good deal of emotional turbulence and exhaustion. When they left for a long-awaited vacation in Alaska, they discontinued all medication so they could enjoy the trip. After their return, they had more than Alaskan gifts to share with the family. In whatever combination of medical help, prayer, and relaxation that took place, Luke and Karen were now expectant parents.

A Child with Destiny

Every baby has a special place in God's heart and plan, but sometimes God indicates to parents that their child is to have a unique future or ministry. This was the case with Roberta, who came to me several years ago when she discovered she was pregnant. Roberta and her husband, Ken, are Christians and had sought God's guidance about a family before they attempted to conceive. Roberta told me that God had spoken to her in a dream before she even knew she was pregnant, assuring her that no matter what happened, He would protect her baby and that their male child would have a special place in God's purpose.

In the first seven months, Roberta's pregnancy seemed normal, but then I noticed that the baby was not growing as it should. When an ultrasound indicated that the baby had intrauterine growth retardation, we began to follow Roberta carefully with special testing. Three weeks later, the baby showed evidence of severe growth restriction caused by insufficient blood flow through the placenta.

Now I had to tell Roberta and Ken that I would have to deliver their baby immediately by cesarean section because of the severe growth retardation. To my amazement, Roberta reminded me of the dream and said, "Don't worry, doctor; my baby will be fine. You just get him out here to us safely!"

Their baby boy weighed just over two pounds at birth, and he required intensive care for almost three months before he could be discharged from the hospital. When he went home, he weighed only five and one-half pounds.

Years later, it is easy to see that God kept His promise. Although he is still young, Roberta's son is brilliant. He has a fantastic memory and is an excellent student. More important, he is a Christian and has been a marvelous witness for Christ at his young age. God always keeps His promises; even when we think that He surely must have messed up, He proves us wrong. As we read earlier in Psalm 139 and Jeremiah 1, God knew each of us when we were in our mother's womb, and He planned our days even before our birth. We should never doubt His sovereignty.

Melissa's Thank-You

After eighteen years in obstetrics, delivering babies is still a thrilling experience for me. The sight of a family rejoicing at the birth of their infant is so rewarding. I use the delivery experience to remind couples of the tremendous privilege they have to be part of such a miraculous process, to be on the receiving end of God's creative power.

I try to pray for each baby with the parents in the delivery room. I know that for some infants, this will be the only prayer ever offered for them. Therefore, I take this opportunity to dedicate the child to God and ask His blessing on the new life.

These experiences at the time of delivery are very rewarding, but an even greater reward is to have some of those children come back to see me when they are older or write me a letter, as Melissa did.

> Dear Dr. Hager,
> I just celebrated my fourteenth birthday. My mother told me that you delivered me. She also told me that you prayed for me right after I was born. I just want you to know that the night of my fourteenth birthday, I accepted Jesus as my personal Savior. Your prayer has been answered.
> Thank you.
> Melissa

four

Coping with Chronic Disease

hen I first saw Vivian as a patient, she was forty-two years old. She and her husband had two children in college. He had an excellent job, she was a homemaker, and they had a comfortable life. She was very active in her church, often spoke at women's groups, and was known to be a woman of prayer. After her initial appointment with me, Vivian let several years go by before making another, and she called for the most recent one only reluctantly, since her husband had lost his job and his health insurance.

When Vivian came in, she told me that she was experiencing such heavy vaginal bleeding that she was continually weak and anemic. Her periods had been heavy for several years, but she had not sought help until she fainted in a store, which frightened her enough to call for an appointment.

As I took her medical history, Vivian told me that for many years she had had an enlarged uterus because of fibroids. Ninety-nine percent of these growths are benign, and they may cause no symptoms at all, or they may cause excessive menstrual bleeding and pelvic pressure or pain. Because of the family's lack of insurance, and because Vivian believed God would take care of her problems, she had ignored her symptoms until now.

When I examined her, I found a mass protruding out of the pelvis up into the abdomen. The most likely explanation for the mass was that her uterus was enlarged by the fibroids. The mass was not tender, and other than the excessive bleeding, Vivian had no symptoms. A check of her hematocrit (the percentage of red blood cells in the blood stream) indicated that she was still very anemic, but a biopsy showed that there was no malignancy in the lining of the uterus.

When Vivian and I talked about her condition, I explained that her uterus was as large as it would be if she were sixteen weeks pregnant. For women with Vivian's condition, surgery to remove the uterus is recommended if the uterus is so large that the ovaries cannot be adequately evaluated by pelvic examination or ultrasound, if the uterus is enlarging rapidly over a short period of time, if the patient has excessive uterine bleeding, or if she has significant pain or pressure on other major organs in the pelvis. If a woman wishes to have more children, we can do a procedure called a myomectomy, in which we make an incision in the uterus and remove the fibroids. But since Vivian had completed her childbearing, it was my opinion that she should have a hysterectomy.

Most women in her situation are pleased that surgery can remove the mass and stop the bleeding, but Vivian was appalled. I assured her that we would do the surgery at a major discount and that I would encourage the hospital to cut its price also, but she adamantly refused. She said, "We will pray about this. I believe God will heal me, and I will not need surgery."

I replied, "Vivian, I believe in divine healing too, but please remember that if the bleeding continues, you are going to become more and more anemic. If you wait too long, you may become severely ill and require a blood transfusion before I can operate on you."

It was two years before I saw her name on my appointment schedule again. I thought, *Good grief, she's probably even more anemic, and the uterus is likely twenty-weeks size by now.* Fibroids may sometimes remain the same size, but in many situations they increase in mass so that the patient becomes more symptomatic. It is very unusual for them to decrease in size.

When I saw Vivian in the exam room, she was pleasant and apologized for not contacting me sooner. "After my pastor prayed for me, I just forgot about the problem," she said.

I asked about her periods, and she indicated that they were now normal in length and amount of flow. She was having no pelvic pain or pressure and had experienced no dizziness or fainting. A check of her hematocrit indicated a marked improvement over the last time I had seen her, and examination revealed only a slightly enlarged uterus. I was astounded and dismissed Vivian to return in six months—hoping that if I was lucky she might come back in a year.

The Prayer of Faith

Vivian had great faith—more than her doctor. I was astounded when I realized that she was miraculously healed. But Vivian recognized her disease, had the faith to believe that God could and would heal her, and then reached out to receive that healing. What a lesson I learned from this woman of faith—a lesson that would enable me to have faith for many other women who came into my office over the years needing the touch of the Master Physician.

It seems that everywhere we look these days, we find something about the connection between prayer and the healing process. Television magazine shows have segments on this, popular magazines and newspapers feature articles, and even medical and scientific journals are giving some space to the subject.

In recent years, research has been done on control groups to see if prayer actually makes a difference in one's health. Debbie Warhola's article, "The Power of Prayer in Healing," covered the issue from both sides, interviewing those who believe that prayer plays an integral role in health and the healing process and others who believe the effect of prayer is simply that of positive thinking. Warhola reported a study of 91,909 persons in rural Maryland who regularly attend church. Compared with a control group of nonchurchgoers, they had 50 percent fewer deaths from heart disease, 74 percent fewer deaths from cirrhosis, 56 percent fewer deaths from emphysema, and 53 percent fewer suicides. Clearly, their lifestyle was important in these differences, since they were more likely to refrain from smoking and excessive drinking. However, the article did not address the subject of faith in God to heal the types of ailments that both study groups would likely have.[1]

What is the significance of faith in obtaining healing? Is faith required in order for healing to occur, and if so, can someone else have faith for you? Is there power in just being prayed for even if you don't know it? Why is one person healed instantaneously, another gradually, and others not healed? Do those who are healed have more faith?

We will talk more about these questions in later chapters, but they came to mind with force as I thought about Vivian. I was also reminded of a woman in the Gospels who had a similar problem.

A Healing Touch

Jewish custom and law dictated that a woman was unclean during her menstrual flow. So the woman we read about in Matthew 9:20–22, Mark 5:25–34, and Luke 8:43–48 took a great chance of being detected when she chose to mingle in the crowds. Had the men present known that for twelve years she had been suffering from heavy bleeding, they would have felt that she contaminated them and would have publicly humiliated her by making her leave. She had apparently counted the cost and felt that she had no other choice than to risk embarrassment.

Because this woman was probably weak and pale as a result of the chronic blood loss, she was desperate to find someone who could help.[2] Unlike Vivian, she had been seeking help for twelve years from a succession of medical people; "she had suffered a great deal under the care of many doctors and had spent all she had, yet instead of getting better she grew worse" (Mark 5:26).

We don't know if she was a religious woman or if there was an element of magic in her thinking. All she knew was that Jesus healed people and didn't send a bill. She was out of money and hope with the establishment, and she had to try something else. If her behavior came across as unacceptable, if she was publicly embarrassed, that was a risk worth taking because of the hope of getting better. She didn't plan to talk to Jesus or ask for anything. She thought, "If I just touch His clothes, I will be healed" (Mark 5:28).

Jesus was in the middle of a crowd when the woman reached out and touched the hem of His cloak. Several others must have touched and jostled Jesus in the crowd, but something about her touch was different. "Immediately her bleeding stopped and she felt in her body that she was freed from her suffering. At once Jesus realized that power had gone out from him. He turned around in the crowd and asked, 'Who touched my clothes?'" (Mark 5:29–30).

Jesus knew healing power had left Him—that power was the Holy Spirit within Him. It remains a mystery how Jesus knew, from all the crowd around Him, that someone had drawn healing power. And what made Him stop and ask who it was? My guess is that He knew, but He was asking her to step out and confirm her healing. It is important to recognize the need for healing and have the faith that healing can occur, but it is also important to confirm the healing when it happens.

The woman realized that this interaction was different from those with all the physicians who had tried to help her. She wasn't walking away heartbroken from yet another medical caregiver, as bad off or worse than before. This time the flow of blood had stopped, and she knew she would not hemorrhage again. Nevertheless, she was frightened when Jesus asked her to identify herself. For just a moment, there was a glimmer of hope that she could escape unnoticed, when the disciples said to Jesus, "You see the people crowding against you . . . and yet you can ask, 'Who touched me?'" (Mark 5:31).

But Jesus wouldn't dismiss it that easily and kept looking around to see who had touched Him. I wonder how long this took, because Jesus waited—He was not going to point her out. She was healed, and if she had chosen not to talk with Him, she could have gone home healed. He respected her privacy and her condition and did not draw attention to her ailment.

Healings don't have to occur in public. God respects your privacy, and He can heal just as effectively when you are alone as in a crowd. But when He asks you to confirm your healing in public, it is important to do so.

Seeing that He was waiting, the woman pressed through the crowd and fell at Jesus' feet, trembling with fear. When she finished telling Him what had happened, Jesus said to her, "Daughter, your faith has healed you. Go in peace and be freed from your suffering" (Mark 5:34). Instead of claiming the credit for the healing, Jesus humbly praised her for her faith. He even called her "Daughter," meaning "child or daughter of Abraham."

It wasn't a magical touch that healed this woman, or the aura of His presence, but the divine touch of God Himself, and Jesus wanted her to understand that. The Creator of the universe was so concerned about her that He allowed His healing power to flow into her body in response to her faith, and then He told her that her trust was crucial in the restoration of her body. Jesus assured her that she was well; she could leave in the emotional peace and the physical confidence that she was cured.

In receiving so graciously the woman who was hemorrhaging, Jesus made another statement about women then and now: "This unclean woman does not contaminate Me. She has a right to approach Me and seek healing, even when I am talking with an official of the synagogue. Women have an important place in society and in My ministry. The faith of this woman made her whole, and her story will encourage women for all ages to believe in Me."

Facing Chronic Disease

The woman in Mark 5 is but one of the many, then and now, suffering from chronic disease. She had particular courage and persistence in her pursuit of healing, especially when we consider how she had been impoverished and made worse physically by her dealings with medical people for twelve years. I have seen many such women in my practice. Perhaps you, too, suffer from a chronic ailment. If so, I want to share with you three attitudes that I often see in these patients.

Resignation. "I'm afflicted with a disease. Since I can't change it, I'll just suffer and try to tolerate it. This is my lot in life. Because I don't want to trouble other people with my problems, I'll try to keep it all inside." Such people usually withdraw and are often depressed.

Repression. "I'm not sick—there is nothing wrong with me. I am not going to talk about illness because if I do, I will have to admit that I am sick. Therefore, I'll go on as if nothing is wrong. I prefer not to address the possibilities of what this disease can do to me." These repressed feelings usually are buried deep in the subconscious, resulting in anxiety and tension. When the disease progresses or suddenly becomes severe, these people are in shock.

Realism. "I'm sick. Lots of people get sick, and I am just one of them. I will not let this get the best of me. I am going to go on with my life in the best way I can." It is important for people like this to remember that God always has their ultimate good at heart.

Women with chronic diseases often want to give up. The pain and suffering are so constant and severe that it seems easier just to lie down and give in to the disease. Their suffering makes it easy to identify with Job, a good and prosperous man who was stricken with the loss of his children and then with a painful and repulsive physical affliction. In *The Message,* Eugene Peterson's translation of the Bible, we read Job's poignant words:

> God alienated my family from me;
>   everyone who knows me avoids me.
> My relatives and friends have all left;
>   houseguests forget I ever existed.
> The servant girls treat me like a bum off the street,
>   look at me like they've never seen me before.
> I call my attendant and he ignores me,
>   ignores me even though I plead with him.

My wife can't stand to be around me anymore.
  I'm repulsive to my family.
Even street urchins despise me;
  when I come out, they taunt and jeer.
Everyone I've ever been close to abhors me;
  my dearest loved ones reject me.
I'm nothing but a bag of bones;
  my life hangs by a thread.

Oh, friends, dear friends, take pity on me.
  God has come down hard on me!
Do you have to be hard on me too?
  Don't you ever tire of abusing me?

If only my words were written in a book—
  better yet, chiseled in stone!
Still, I know that God lives—the One who gives me back
    my life—
and eventually he'll take his stand on earth.
And I'll see him—even though I get skinned alive!—
  see God myself, with my very own eyes.
Oh, how I long for that day!

Job 19:13–27

Refusing to Give Up

Hazel and Charlotte are two women with chronic ailments who did not give up. They continued to believe, as Job did, that in spite of what happened to them, God lives and is the One who gives them back their lives.

Hazel was a young woman with end-stage renal disease. *End-stage* means that the disease was severe and would ultimately be fatal unless she received a transplant. She went to kidney dialysis three times a week for five years. Although she was aware of her poor prognosis and obviously didn't enjoy having to go to the renal clinic so often, you wouldn't have known this to talk with her. She always had a smile and a kind word for everyone. She never complained, even when she felt horrible. She could have been on disability but decided she wanted to make a contribution to society in spite of her infirmity, and so she developed a business that she could run from her home. She remained active in her church and became an advocate for improved facilities for the impaired in her community. Hazel felt fortunate that she was alive, and she wanted to give something of herself to others.

Charlotte is a young woman with multiple sclerosis.[3] When I saw her, she was seriously ill, walking with the use of a walker, experiencing atrophy of her muscles, and having difficulty seeing. She easily could have given up and allowed herself to become more and more dissipated. Instead, she remains as active as she possibly can. She cares for her children, is involved in church, paints water-color scenes, and writes beautiful poetry. She spends time calling others who are sick and writes letters to bereaved families. What a ministry her life is—a great encouragement to those who are tempted to allow their disease to get the best of them.

The Day Barbara Was Healed

During her high school years Barbara Cummiskey began to develop symptoms that affected her coordination to the extent that other students joked behind her back that she was drunk. Despite several series of tests, her doctor did not positively diagnose Barbara until 1970, by which time she was in college. She was told that she had multiple sclerosis (MS) and that there was almost nothing that could be done except to hope her case was a mild one.

Over the following years, Barbara's MS went through cycles of worsening and then stabilizing. She was able to continue with college and also to work until 1978, when she was in a wheelchair and needed oxygen every day. A trip to the Mayo Clinic yielded no hope; the doctors there told her to pray.

This was not a new idea to Barbara—she had committed her life to the Lord as a child, and during her teenage years had grown much closer to Him. As her disease became more disabling, Pastor Bailie from the Wheaton Wesleyan Church was a constant support to her. He was the one who convinced her that she needed a goal, a purpose, and she decided that hers would be to grow in faith.

As Barbara lost physical health, she prayed that God would give her spiritual health. He showed her that there was something she could do in her search for this health— to pray for others.

While Barbara was deepening her trust in God and growing in her knowledge of His Word, her physical health deteriorated and she was technically blind. In 1980 one lung collapsed, and Barbara had a tracheostomy to increase her oxygen supply. Her parents had already talked with the local hospice in anticipation of the time that Barbara would need their care.

Early in June of 1981, Pastor Bailie visited Barbara and thought that would be the last time he would see her alive. Sunday, June 7, was her sister's birthday, and Barbara wanted to be with her mother in the kitchen to at least think she was helping with the birthday cake. Her twisted hands could manage no more than a few turns with the spoon before she had to wheel back to her room and get into bed.

Later that afternoon, two friends arrived for a visit. As the three of them talked, Barbara heard another voice from behind her say, "My child, get up and walk!" Startled, she realized that her friends had not heard the words. She said to them, "Joyce, Angela, God just spoke to me.

He said to get up and walk. I heard Him! Go and get my
family!"

As they ran to find her parents, Barbara took action. She
pulled the oxygen tube from her throat, removed the brace
from her arm and jumped out of bed to stand on legs that
hadn't held her for five years. She looked at her hands and
saw that they were no longer curled. Her legs were filled out
and her twisted feet were now flat on the floor. She started
to walk out of the room just as her mother came in. Her dad
was next, and he took her to the family room where she
showed all of them how she could navigate normally.

Barbara's church had a Sunday evening service, and she
determined to go. She entered the back of the sanctuary,
just as Pastor Bailie asked if anyone had other announce-
ments. The young woman he thought he would never see
alive again walked down the aisle! Barbara threw her arms
into the air, praising God for her healing. She proceeded
to describe her miraculous healing to the speechless congregation, and together, Barbara and these fellow believers shed tears of joy at God's marvelous healing touch!

The next day Barbara called her doctor and then went
to his office where he greeted her in astonishment. After
three hours of tests, he shook his head and said that he
found no sign of MS and that Barbara should stop taking
her medications. Also, both her lungs were now functioning normally. Another doctor who had performed
surgeries on her concurred with the opinion and talked
about "the good hand of God in her life."

Today Barbara is a wife and mother and ministers with
her pastor husband in their Virginia church. Her story
appeared in *Guideposts* in April of 1985. She said:

> I don't know why God healed me. I don't believe I "earned"
> or "deserved" a healing any more than I "deserved" MS.
> I only know that on the morning of June 7, 1981, I felt
> good about myself—mentally, emotionally and spiritually

well. Through my prayer life, I was a busy, active member
of the human family—not running or jumping or even
walking like most people, but not separated from them by
bitterness, self-pity or despair. My mind and spirit were
healthy and whole. And then, God made my body whole
too.[4]

God never promised us a life of ease, but He does promise
us the resources to survive whatever the world can throw
our way. He also promises us healing if we will believe. Perhaps that healing will not occur just as we expect, but there
will be healing enough to allow us to minister to others if
we will look for opportunities.

Satan would love to defeat us and convince us that God
has abandoned us when we become ill, especially when
we face chronic disease. But God has promised that He
will never leave us, and He gives us the Holy Spirit to
strengthen and sustain us in our times of greatest need.
We can be certain that He will be there.

five

Misused Women

When Jean strolled into my office, she was strikingly attired in skintight slacks and a shocking-pink sweater. Her appearance told me that she was a woman in desperate need of attention. As I began to take her medical history, what she told me confirmed my suspicions.

Jean was born in Mississippi, where her father was a salesman. His frequent business trips gave him opportunity to meet many women, and his compulsive infidelity threatened and finally destroyed his marriage. When Jean was only five, she and her sister moved with their mother to Tennessee. Because her father never contacted the family, Jean was denied the love and attention she should have received from him.

Jean's mother was extremely possessive, insecure, and overprotective. She attempted to maintain control of her daughters and prevent them from making friends, especially male friends. She was also very suspicious of their activities whenever they were away from her. "Mother tried to make up for Daddy's absence in her life by clinging to us. It wasn't just an effort to keep us away from guys. When we wanted to spend the night at a girlfriend's house, she would accuse us of loving our girlfriends more than we did her. She was always shaming and blaming us: 'You have to make me happy; you have to stay with me and please me.'"

When she was nineteen, Jean broke loose from her mother's control and began to be sexually active in a series of short-term relationships. She told me, "I know now that I was trying to find a substitute for my absent father and to rebel against my clinging mother." Because she gave no thought to the possible consequences of her choices, Jean was shocked when she discovered that she was twenty weeks pregnant. By the time she considered abortion, she was twenty-three weeks along and could not find a clinic that would terminate the pregnancy. She felt she had no alternative but to carry the pregnancy to term.

"I gave birth to a healthy baby boy but then felt desperate about how I could support him. The only solution I could see was to marry the man I assumed was the father, even though it could have been one of several. He said he loved me so much that he would marry me regardless of whether he was the father. The marriage didn't last long though, and within a year I was back in the dating scene.

"I returned to school to pursue a degree. In a music class I met Roger, who was ten years older than me. I found that he met some of my needs for a father, because I assumed he was mature. He fell in love with me and divorced his wife to marry me. In the next three years, I had two more children."

Unfortunately, Roger was very much like her father in his infidelities and eventually left the family, depriving Jean and her three children of the love and support they needed from him. Because Roger made no attempt to care for the family, Jean was forced to go on welfare.

This indignity, plus everything else that had happened in her short life, plunged her self-esteem to its lowest point. She felt condemned by society and was frequently confused and depressed. Just seeing a husband and wife together with their children seemed to mock her and intensified the grief she tried to keep hidden deep within her spirit. When she thought things couldn't get any worse, Jean began to experience some puzzling physical symptoms. She was frightened by the pain and discomfort, so she sought help from a public health clinic. They diagnosed human papilloma virus (HPV) and precancerous change of the cervix.[1] Jean underwent laser treatment for the HPV and cervical dysplasia and was cured, but five years later she still harbored deep-seated hate toward Roger for infecting her.

As Jean told me the details of her tragic story, the hardened spirit of this wounded woman began to break open. Bitter anger toward her father, her mother, and God poured from her in a raging stream. Jean despised all men because of what she had suffered at the hands of a few. As I listened, I silently prayed that the love of God, which Jean had never experienced, would reach her through me.

"Jean," I said, "when a person exhibits addictive or abusive behavior, you can count on the fact that he was abused as a child or lived with an addict. Do you know anything about Roger's parents?"

"I know that his father was an alcoholic and that he was very hard on Roger. He told me once that he always felt he was the one who had to hold the family together when things were going badly. He felt responsible for the welfare of everyone else."

I told Jean, "Roger's desire to hold the family together is a typical codependent response of a child of an alcoholic. Your husband wanted to love but didn't know how, because he had never seen it demonstrated in his home. He thought that loving someone meant possessing and controlling. He saw the damaging effects of alcohol and so resisted it, but instead, he became addicted to sex. I know it is hard after what he did to you, but if you can put it in the perspective of how he was abandoned emotionally, you may develop some sympathy for him."

As Jean's anger spent itself, cleansing tears began to spill from her eyes. We talked together about the Spirit of Truth, who could ultimately set her free from the bondages of her life. I explained that true intimacy of spirit can occur only with the Holy Spirit, who will never let you down as people often do. As we talked, Jean began to realize that she was as victimized by her own unwillingness to admit to and deal with her anger and her own sexual addictions as she was by the cruelties of the many men who had crossed her downhill path.

The Woman at the Well

Jean's story reminded me of the Samaritan woman Jesus met beside a well. This woman also felt condemned and rejected by society, and with more reason than Jean had. The Jews regarded all Samaritans as mongrels—unclean people who had committed the unforgivable sin of intermarrying with foreigners in the past and producing a mixed race. Because orthodox Jews prized racial purity, they would not even cross the road to help a Samaritan. Whenever possible, they avoided traveling through Samaria. Their differences were long and bitter, dating back hundreds of years, during which the Jews and Samaritans had developed different religious and cultural ways, with each group claiming it possessed the truth of God.

To be a Samaritan and a woman was to be under a double curse. Women of any race or creed were considered chattel to first-century men. Their primary value was in their capacity to produce male heirs and to carry out the duties of running a home. To have any sort of contact with a woman who had recently had sexual intercourse or who was menstruating was to risk contamination, since that woman was considered ceremonially unclean. So an observant Jewish male would not talk to any woman in public, because he could not be certain that she was ritually clean.

We need to remember that Jesus was raised in an orthodox home. He also was a teacher—a rabbi. For Him to be seen speaking to a woman in public was unthinkable. For Him to go out of His way to talk at length with a Samaritan woman was beyond belief. But the Son of God came to fulfill the law, not to be bound to man-made customs and rituals. Jesus chose to journey through Samaria to testify to this reality. He had an appointment of eternal importance to keep with a certain Samaritan woman, even though she didn't know it (John 4:4–42).

In the heat of the sixth hour, or noontime, Jesus and His weary disciples came to the town of Sychar, about thirty miles north of Jerusalem. As the disciples went off to buy food in town, Jesus sat down beside Jacob's well,[2] for He was very tired from the journey. Can you see Him there—hot, thirsty, dusty, and tired, leaning against the well, wiping sweat from His brow? Then He saw a woman approaching to draw water.

Wells such as this were usually meeting places for the women of the town who came to draw water for their families. Yet this Samaritan woman came alone. Many Bible students have thought she was trying to avoid the other women and perhaps escape their criticism and rejection. She was not like them—she had had five husbands and lived with a man to whom she was not married.

Jesus seemed to ignore the woman's ostracism. He asked her, "Will you give me a drink?" (John 4:7). He who could

have called on the angels of heaven to meet His need chose
to ask this foreign woman for water.

Instead of turning away from Him or meeting His
request with silence, the woman replied, "You are a Jew
and I am a Samaritan woman. How can you ask me for
a drink?" (John 4:9). She was incredulous that this Jewish
man would be so brazen as to speak to her, much less
request a favor.

Jesus heard her reply, but He also understood her heart.
As He asked her to minister to His physical need, He
wanted to minister to her spiritual need—to give her the
living water that would quench her inner thirst. She had
come to meet a physical need—to draw water for herself
and her family—but she soon forgot about that as she
entered into the most amazing conversation she had ever
had. Jesus did not answer her questions directly, and yet
He led her to the answer she had been seeking all her life—
someone to deeply know and understand her and still
accept her for who she was and who she could be.

In Jesus' words to the Samaritan woman, women today
also can find answers to their deepest questions. Jesus
talked with the Samaritan woman with respect, compassion, sensitivity, and understanding. He did not speak to
her in a condescending manner as so many men do to
women (and doctors can be the worst offenders). Instead
He spoke in a way that respected her intellect and assumed
she would understand Him. With spiritual sensitivity, He
drew on their common religious background. He spoke of
her inner feelings of dryness—something we have all experienced at times.

Because Jesus knew the inner workings of her soul as
only God can, He realized that her desperation, her loneliness and despair, her anxiety and guilt had created a
hardened exterior that was now cracking from a lack of
refreshing water within. He knew that she craved true satisfaction in her relationships, but she was so broken and

shattered that she could not establish lasting relationships in which she could love and be loved.

As Jesus offered her living water that would forever quench her inner thirst, she began to understand that He was speaking of eternal forgiveness and salvation. He had promised, "Everyone who drinks this water will be thirsty again, but whoever drinks the water I give him will never thirst. Indeed, the water I give him will become in him a spring of water welling up to eternal life" (John 4:13–14).

When the woman asked for that spring of water, Jesus said, "Go, call your husband and come back" (John 4:16). When she replied that she had no husband, Jesus told her that he knew about her five husbands and her current man. This convinced her that He was a prophet, but she had a defensive tactic to shift the focus from her sins. She wanted to discuss the different places where the Jews and Samaritans worshiped. Jesus answered this concern but then told her, "God is spirit, and his worshipers must worship in spirit and in truth" (John 4:24).

Like all of us, the Samaritan woman could not truly worship until she was honest with God about who she was and confessed her sins. Jesus' mention of her current live-in situation indicates that infidelity had played a major role in her life. Like Jean, this woman of Samaria must have been deeply hurt by men. As a result she seemed unable to engage in lasting relationships. She undoubtedly had low self-esteem and probably experienced severe feelings of guilt for her indiscretions.

What a relief it must have been to meet a man who was interested in who she was and how she felt, and who treated her with respect. Jesus teaches men today a great lesson: When we communicate with women, we should affirm them, talk to them as equals, and show concern for their real needs.

When the disciples returned, they were astounded to find Jesus talking with a woman, but she probably didn't notice, since she left her water jar and ran back to the village to tell her neighbors about this amazing person she had met. She had gone to the well that day feeling downtrodden, lonely, and sinful; she returned to her village as a forgiven witness to the love of God. She was so convincing, so changed, that people who didn't even respect her followed her back to see this Man who had challenged her.

When the villagers talked with Jesus at the well, they were so impressed that they invited Him to stay with them so that they, too, might receive the living water. He stayed two days, and many of the people became believers. Through the testimony of an immoral woman, many people found the purity of forgiveness and the reality of a personal relationship with the God they thought they knew, but whose ways they had forsaken. Jesus' appointment with one woman on a hot day in Samaria forever changed the lives of many.

Poor Choices

The woman at the well was not unique. Jean and many other modern women live with the consequences of similar poor choices. But Jesus offers a second chance by extending His love and forgiveness to them.

Beth was an attractive young woman who seemed embarrassed to be in my office. She had been divorced for over a year and had recently decided to reenter the dating scene. Unfortunately, the man she became interested in withheld some vital information until they had gone out several times. He failed to tell her that he was married and he might have an infection that could have been passed on to her. Although she had no symptoms yet, Beth wanted to be screened for chlamydia.[3]

In talking with her, I asked if this man was a steady partner. She replied, "Well, I've gone out with several guys since I started dating again, but he is the only one for the past two months."

"Beth, I don't want to embarrass you, but in determining who we may need to screen, I have to know if you have slept with all these men."

"No . . . I mean yes . . . yes, I slept with them." Suddenly she began to cry. "I really didn't want to," she sobbed, "but they seemed to expect it of me, probably because I'm divorced. It is such a different scene now than when I was dating before. Everybody seems to expect sex."

As we talked more, I emphasized that if she didn't take pride in herself and protect her own body, no one else would. She indicated that she would like to stop her sexual activity, but she didn't want to stay at home alone all the time. She said, "I really want to do what is right, but it is just so hard these days."

Then Beth said, "Dr. Hager, I don't think I will ever be able to look my family in the eye again, after all this, and I don't think I can ever be forgiven for what I have done."

I replied, "Beth, your sin is no greater than that of anyone else. You need to read some stories in the New Testament about women who were involved in adultery, especially the woman brought to Jesus by some religious leaders in John 8 and the Samaritan woman at the well in John 4. If you seek Jesus' forgiveness and confess your sins, He will forgive you. He assures us of this in 1 John 1:9: 'If we confess our sins, he is faithful and just and will forgive us our sins and purify us from all unrighteousness.'

"You are in your current situation because you have made some poor choices based on what you want. It is important that you learn the principle of paradox taught in the Bible—in giving up yourself you gain; in laying down what you crave, you find what you thought you would lose (Matt. 10:39). Jesus accepts you just as you are.

All you have to do is place your life in His hands and let Him shape and refine you into the special individual He created you to be."

By then the tears were streaming down Beth's face. I asked if she would mind if we prayed. "No, please do." I prayed a simple prayer, asking God to forgive her and enable her to remain abstinent until she remarried. Then I asked if she wanted to pray for forgiveness. She hesitated and then sobbed, "I'm sorry. I really am." That was enough. God knew her heart.

A year later, I received a card from Beth thanking me for being a vehicle of God's love and telling me that she had remained abstinent. Yes, God can and does forgive, no matter what the sin.

Childhood Abuse

Nancy was twenty-eight when she came to my office complaining of irregular menstrual periods, headaches, and diarrhea. I initiated a routine evaluation, including an examination and laboratory work, all of which came back normal. Since the most frequent cause of this type of bleeding in younger women is hormonal, and because stress is a frequent cause of the hormonal dysfunction, headaches, and diarrhea, I asked Nancy if she was under significant stress. She replied, "Dr. Hager, I have been seeing doctors for ten years with various problems and have wished that someone would ask me that question. I know it sounds strange, but I just couldn't admit it myself."

When I asked her to tell me about it, her story slowly unfolded: "I was raised in Africa where my parents served as missionaries. We children were sent two hundred miles away to a mission boarding school. We had to go to the headmaster for individual academic reviews as well as when we did anything wrong. When I was thirteen, the headmaster began using these visits to kiss me on the neck or touch my breasts. If I tried to move away, he insisted that I sit still. Sometimes he made me sit on his lap. He kept me silent by threats of my expulsion or the possible expulsion of my parents from the field if I ever told anyone, which would have publicly humiliated me, separated me from all my friends, and greatly disappointed my parents. There were times when I wanted to be sent home to escape the headmaster, but I was afraid of how my parents would react.

"Dr. Hager, this same man led chapel services during the week and preached on Sundays. I couldn't believe what he—supposedly a man of God—was doing to me, and I began to wonder if I somehow caused him to think he could treat me that way."

I asked Nancy if the other girls ever talked about his behavior with them. She replied, "No, and I didn't say anything to them, because I was afraid they would think I was dirty. I was so upset that it affected my grades, and I lost a lot of weight. I was in conflict—confused, angry, guilty, and at the same time feeling very hypocritical.

"I have never been able to tell anyone about this before, but I am so desperate now that I have to talk about it. I have developed a total lack of trust of men, and I have no self-esteem at all. I'm afraid if my female friends knew about this, they would think that I am cheap and disgusting. And I am unable to date, because I can't believe a man could love me for who I really am."

Taking a deep breath, I tried to maintain control over the extreme anger I felt at this man who had so horribly affected Nancy's life. After a moment I told her, "Nancy, it is vitally important that you get into a counseling program immediately. You are not responsible for what happened to you—you were a victim. The headmaster had a major problem with sexual addiction and probably damaged many other girls too. I can refer you to a wonderful Christian counselor."

I wanted to pray with Nancy, but before I could suggest this, she asked me, "Why do you think God allowed this to happen to me as a Christian?"

I hesitated for a moment and then said, "Nancy, I don't know why bad things happen to good people, but I do know that God loves you and was deeply troubled by what happened to you. He will help you to recover from this and will enable you to love and even to forgive again."

"No, I don't think I will ever be able to forgive him for what he has done to me!"

I didn't press the issue with her, but I felt confident that God would bring healing to Nancy, including the capacity to forgive at some point. I then prayed for her emotional and physical healing and that God would bring friends into her life who could love and encourage her.

In the months that followed, Nancy stayed with the counseling and did well. Her periods became regular, and her other stress-related symptoms decreased. She met a young man who became a real friend to her, and then a more serious relationship developed that eventually led to marriage.

Drinking the Living Water

Two thousand years after the Samaritan woman met Jesus, Jean, Beth, and Nancy opened themselves to the living water that Jesus offers. Like the woman by the well, they have seen their lives restored by the Master's love and forgiveness as He touched them at their point of deepest need. They have experienced restoration as only Jesus can restore and fulfillment as only He can fulfill.

For these women, salvation began with a willingness to admit their sin or, in Nancy's case, being sinned against, which had become a barrier between them and God. But for them, as for all of us, salvation does not end with an initial drink of living water. After giving them the gift of true repentance and trust, Jesus began to show them the way to wholeness. They awakened to their need of God when they experienced the reality of God's unconditional love.

No matter how bad your situation, how deep or long-lived your sins, Jesus waits at the place where you are drawing water, trying to find something to nourish the inner drought of your existence. He offers you acceptance, forgiveness, and a depth of love you will not fully believe until you fully receive it. He who knows you most fully loves you most completely—right where you are today. Jesus Christ can transform and restore your life in the moment when you choose to receive His offer of living water.

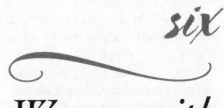

Women with
Wounded Hearts

i did a double take as I looked at the next name on my patient chart. Never in my life had I had a consultation with a Sparkle.

I knocked on the exam room door and entered. Seated on the table was a young woman with streaked blonde hair, dangling earrings, excessive makeup, and more rings than I had ever seen on two hands—at least fifteen! She smiled briefly, but that greeting was quickly replaced with a frown. Sparkle's eyes did not match her name; they conveyed a deep sadness and lack of trust.

She was in my office because I had recently treated one of her friends for a gynecological problem. Sparkle was complaining of abdominal and pelvic pain and abnormal vaginal discharge during the past week. She had been unable to work and said that her pain was becoming progressively worse.

After the examination, I explained to Sparkle that she had pelvic inflammatory disease (PID), a sexually trans-

mitted infection of the uterus and fallopian tubes.[1] She
would have to enter the hospital to be treated with intra-
venous antibiotics. I asked her, "I know that you're hurting from this infection, Sparkle, but are you okay otherwise?" When she didn't respond, I continued, "I realize
that you don't know me well enough as a physician to
trust me, but if you aren't safe or if you are hurting emotionally, my staff and I would like to help you."

Sparkle said nothing, but her head dropped and the
tears began to run down her cheeks, smearing her thick
makeup. I waited for a while and then asked, "Do you
know why you are so depressed?"

Sparkle began her story and continued it intermittently
over the five days she spent in the hospital. She grew up
in the Midwest, the only child of middle-class parents.
When she was seven, her father left home for another
woman. Sparkle told me, "I remember the day he left like
it was yesterday. He said it was best for all of us, that he
loved me, but that he and my mom had problems they
just couldn't resolve. I grabbed his leg as he walked out
the door and clung to the cuff of his pants as he tried to
pull away. Sobbing hysterically, I begged him not to go,
but he unwrapped my fingers from his pants and said,
'I'm sorry, Honey, but I have to go.' I could hardly breathe.
It felt as if my life were coming to an end."

I have found a pattern of abandonment among women
who were hurt for a lifetime by absent fathers who chose
work or another woman over their own families, and Sparkle
was no exception. She continued, "I made a vow to myself
right then to never trust another man, to never get close
enough to be hurt like that again. I would never reveal
myself or give myself to anyone." Then Sparkle began to cry.

"I blamed my mother for causing my dad to leave and
never felt close to her, so when I was eighteen, I moved
away from home. I found a job as a waitress in Kentucky.

Lots of guys came in regularly, and they were nice to me and gave good tips and compliments. One of them asked me out, and I decided to go.

"It turned out that he ran a club for men—a strip joint. He asked me to work there waiting tables, and he offered me good money. After I had worked for him several months, he convinced me to try dancing at the club. I had always enjoyed dancing, and so I agreed. Although I was embarrassed and uncomfortable at first, I quickly found out that I could have control over men and leave them wanting me, rather than vice versa."

Because she was encouraged to mingle with the club's regulars, Sparkle eventually became sexually involved with some of them. She still felt that she had power over the men, since she was leaving them rather than the other way around. However, the consequences of her lifestyle began to catch up with her as she contracted one infection after another—chlamydia, herpes, and human papilloma virus. She soon realized that she wasn't in control but was being used by men in her subconscious attempt to get back at her father. Every time one of them got out of bed to leave, she saw her father walking out the door.

As Sparkle went on with her heartbreaking story, I was reminded of a woman Jesus met who was generally known in her town as a sinner, but whom Jesus saw through eyes of love.

The Woman with the Alabaster Jar

Lush gardens around a fountain were a likely setting for the dinner party given by Simon, a wealthy Pharisee. Among the guests was a young Galilean rabbi. Good manners would have demanded that Simon offer his guest a welcoming hand on the shoulder, the kiss of peace, and a pitcher of cool water to cleanse His dusty feet. But Simon did none of this for Jesus, nor did he place the traditional drop of rose oil on Jesus' forehead.

When the meal was served, Jesus reclined at the table with the other guests, perhaps wondering why He had been invited. Possibly Simon was curious why so many people were excited by the teachings and miracles of this carpenter-become-rabbi from Nazareth. Simon certainly did not want to learn from Him—Simon considered himself a good man. As a student of the Law and the Prophets, he doubtless kept all the commandments.

Whenever a rabbi was a guest in a large home, it was the custom that other people were free to come in and listen to what he said. As Simon and his guests were eating, a young woman entered the courtyard carrying an alabaster jar. Those who lived nearby all knew her—she was the sinner of the neighborhood. As she came in, she must have seen the looks of amazement and heard the snickers and comments, but she passed through the tables until she stood behind Jesus. She had heard Him teach, and His words had pierced her wounded heart. When she found out Jesus would be at Simon's home, she had quickly made her way to the house.

The woman had brought along a delicate flask of perfume with one purpose in mind—to pour it on Jesus' feet. Trembling as she came close to Him, she unashamedly began to weep, and her tears fell on His feet. Without a word, ignoring the shocked faces and gasps of the dinner guests, she loosened her hair (an action considered terribly immodest in her day) and began to wipe His feet with her dark tresses. Then she kissed His feet and poured her perfume on them.

Can you imagine how many tears it took to actually wash the feet of Jesus? This woman wasn't just crying; she must have been sobbing out the agony she felt over her sin. Tears ran down her cheeks, washed over the feet of Jesus, and cleansed away the dust of the road.

Why would a hardened woman of the streets cry so easily?[2] Perhaps she had cried herself to sleep on many lonely nights. Maybe she had cried in pain when she was sexually misused by the men to whom she had sold her body. On this night though, she was pouring out to Jesus a lifetime of pent-up guilt and anguish.

When Simon the Pharisee saw what was happening, he was disturbed that a rabbi would allow such a woman to approach Him in this way. He said to himself, "If this man were a prophet, he would know who is touching him and what kind of woman she is—that she is a sinner" (Luke 7:39).

Hearing the question of Simon's heart, Jesus told him a story about two men who were in debt to a certain lender. One man owed him five hundred silver coins, the other fifty. Since they were both unable to pay, the lender canceled the debts. Who then would love the lender more?

Simon responded, "I suppose the one who had the bigger debt canceled."

After telling him that he was correct, Jesus said,

> "Do you see this woman? I came into your house. You did not give me any water for my feet, but she wet my feet with her tears and wiped them with her hair. You did not give me a kiss, but this woman, from the time I entered, has not stopped kissing my feet. You did not put oil on my head, but she has poured perfume on my feet. Therefore, I tell you, her many sins have been forgiven—for she loved much. But he who has been forgiven little loves little."
> Then Jesus said to her, "Your sins are forgiven."
> Luke 7:44–48

In allowing this woman's display of great contrition for her sins, Jesus encouraged her to be in touch with her deepest feelings and aspirations. In forgiving her sins, He lifted her up to the possibility of worship and praise of her Creator. He does the same for you and me.

I remember a day in a Washington, D.C., hotel room when God spoke to me in a definite way, indicating that unless I repented of my sin and confessed it, He could go no deeper in His relationship with me. For several hours, I battled with God and resisted doing what He was asking; but finally, when I realized that I had to do this or lose my opportunity to grow in my relationship with God and my family, I fell on my knees and the tears began to flow in an unceasing stream. I didn't think they would ever stop.

When we realize that the God of the universe has taken such note of us that He came into the world to die for us so that our sins can be forgiven and forgotten, our gratitude opens the floodgates and our tears flow freely in recognition of such a Savior.

Risking Rejection

The sinful woman who came to Jesus must have considered the risks and counted the cost of being further embarrassed, ridiculed, criticized, and misunderstood before she decided to enter Simon's house that night. The only question that remained was whether Jesus would also reject her. What if He found her to be too unclean, too forward, too damaging to His ministry, or too unimportant to be considered? Yet her burden was great, and her desire for cleansing was profound. Her need to express her love to the Master was so consuming that she risked everything to seek the forgiveness she needed from the Giver of Life. And in going to Jesus, she finally found a Man who really understood her and accepted her for who she was rather than for what she could do for Him. Jesus expected nothing in return; He would never use her.

Sparkle also took risks in her search for physical healing. She finally revealed something about her inner pain, which had led her in such an unhealthy direction. As she recognized how and why she behaved as she did, Sparkle was able to admit the anger and resentment that was eating her up inside. In trying to get back at her father by hurting others, she constantly hurt herself and destroyed every relationship.

Today Sparkle is a changed person. As she got into counseling, she experienced emotional healing over time. She also came to realize that God really loves her and that He is the only one with whom she can find true soul intimacy. In her desperation, Sparkle had nothing to lose and everything to gain by believing in the One who said to her as well as to the woman with the alabaster jar, "Your faith has saved you; go in peace."

Crying for Compassion

Rachelle also had to expose her inner pain before she found true healing. I first met her in the emergency room of a hospital where I was the ob/gyn doctor on call. She lay on the exam table in a fetal position, moaning and complaining of lower abdominal pain.

As I gathered Rachelle's history, I discovered she had seen several gynecologists before and had been diagnosed with chlamydia, a sexually transmitted disease, which had resulted in pelvic inflammatory disease (PID). I thought this would turn out to be PID again, even though she insisted that she had not been sexually active in recent months. The examination was difficult because she was

moaning so much, but I could find no obvious site of tenderness. She had no fever, and all her laboratory findings
were normal. Because I was still concerned, I scheduled a
laparoscopic evaluation to see if we could find what was
wrong internally, but even this showed no abnormality.
After the procedure, I told Rachelle and her family that
I could find no cause for her pain. She immediately began
sobbing and said that I didn't take her seriously or believe
that she was truly in pain. I explained that pain is pain,
if that is what the patient is feeling. Often we can find a
physical cause, but sometimes we cannot.

Rachelle's parents asked to speak to me privately. They
told me their daughter had made frequent visits to doctors' offices and emergency rooms for similar complaints.
Never had anyone suggested that her problem might be
emotionally based—a cry for attention and compassion.
I discovered that Rachelle had been rejected by her
boyfriend, she never had experienced a quality relationship with her father, and her self-esteem was very low. She
internalized her emotional distress, resulting in very real
pain for which we could find no physical cause. Reluctantly, Rachelle agreed to see a counselor and also to ini-
tiate a program of withdrawal from prescription narcotics.

Some months later, Rachelle's mother called me to say
that her daughter was much improved. She was off pain
medication, was spending time with her family, and was
also making new friends. Rachelle's desperation had led
her to cry out for help in a way that is not unusual for
abused or frightened young women—internalizing the
emotional distress and developing pain in some area of
the body. Through counseling, she was finally able to
admit that her medical complaints were really a cry for
emotional help. Her desire to have people pamper and
cater to her every need was not a valid way to try to meet
her true needs. She had been abusing those she said she
loved, by forcing them to care for her. As she grew emo-

tionally, she began to love herself and to respect the real Rachelle, rather than the false self she had been presenting to others.

Caring for His Sheep

When Jesus' forgiveness dramatically changes a sinner's life, gratitude is a natural response. Each of us finds ways to show our thankfulness for God's grace. But I was humbled by the sacrificial servanthood of one woman who truly followed Jesus' command to feed His sheep.

A thirty-year-old mother of three young children, Cassandra was referred to me by her family physician. It was easy to misjudge her by her appearance: She was not very attractive; her clothes were in need of mending; and her hair wanted some attention. Her husband was a construction worker who was away long hours and left the childrearing to Cassandra.

As I took her history, she hesitantly told me about herself. "I've been having pain in my lower abdomen for several weeks. It hurts when I bend over or lift anything heavy."

"Have you had abnormal bleeding?" I asked her.

"No. My periods have been normal, but this one is two weeks late."

My examination revealed a large ovarian cyst that was tender to the touch. I told her that because of its size and her age, surgery would be necessary.

"Dr. Hager, I can't have surgery." Her head dropped, and her face showed dismay.

"What do you mean?" I asked.

"Well, I have three children to care for, plus I help two single mothers with their children by getting clothes for them from the shelter, taking them to school, and fixing

some of their meals. If I'm not there, they won't be cared
for."

Although this woman was stretched to provide for her
own children adequately, she was sacrificially providing
for four other children. I asked her, "Why do you do this?"

"I have to. You see, when I gave my life to Jesus, I was
transformed from a horrible sinner into His child. He made
a completely new woman of me. I heard Him say to me,
'Since I've done this for you, I want you to go now and feed
My sheep.' The only sheep I know to care for are children.
I do this to show my gratitude to Jesus for saving me."

I was embarrassed. God has blessed me, and I give back
to His work without reservation, but this woman was giving all she had. She was being the hands and feet of Christ
to others, even though many in her situation expect some
assistance for themselves. I said to her, "Cassandra, you are
a blessing to those children, and God will bless you for it."

Without hesitation, she replied, "He already has!"

Cassandra convinced me to observe the cyst for another
four weeks so that she could avoid immediate surgery.
Sure enough, the cyst resolved, and she did not require
treatment. She was pleased, and the children—God's
lambs—were cared for.

As I considered Cassandra's ministry, I thought again
of the woman at Simon's house who had been saved from
a life of sin by the forgiveness of God Himself and who in
humility offered herself in service to her Master. I had to
ask myself if I was grateful enough for my salvation to
wash feet, feed the poor, clothe the naked, or visit the
lonely in thankfulness to Jesus.

I was also reminded of Sparkle's words when she told
me about her father: "I made a vow to myself right then
that I would never get close enough to be hurt like that
again. I would never reveal myself or give myself to anyone." I thought of how we all wall off areas of our lives to

protect ourselves from further hurt. When someone hurts us, abandons us, or embarrasses us, we decide that we will do whatever it takes never to let that happen again, making subconscious vows to guard the most vulnerable parts of ourselves.

These vows may lead us to behaviors that are evil or socially unacceptable before we experience forgiveness or that are overly self-protective even after we have come to know Christ's love. Yet, He is always ready to help us denounce those vows and to break down those walls that are really barriers to the inner healing God wants to do in our lives. He desires to care for our wounds, and He will, as we are willing to open ourselves to Him and to His loving ministry in our lives.

seven

Waiting for God's Perfect Timing

*i*n the Gospel of John, we find the amazing story of Jesus raising His friend Lazarus from the dead. Our focus in the story is usually on the restoration of life to Lazarus. However, restoration also occurred on that miraculous day in the grieving sisters, Martha and Mary.

Both John (11:1–44; 12:1–11) and Luke (10:38–42) tell us about this family of Bethany—a brother and two sisters living together and often sharing their home with Jesus and His disciples. When Lazarus became ill, the sisters sent messengers to Jesus to tell Him of His good friend's condition. Jesus' response was certainly not like an old-time general practitioner.

Dr. J. S. Williams was one of those family practitioners who impacted the lives of many patients. His example of dedicated service inspired me to go into the field of medicine. No matter what the time of day, condition of the weather, or how he felt, Dr. Williams went out to see patients who could not come to his office. Even when it

95

was very inconvenient, Dr. Williams would come to the assistance of a patient or family at a moment's notice. His compassionate and caring attitude was an inspiration to me in my youth.

In contrast, Jesus didn't stop what He was doing and immediately travel to Bethany. He delayed so that by the time He and the disciples finally arrived in Bethany, Lazarus had already been buried for four days, and his sisters and friends were grieving.

Practical, efficient Martha met Jesus first with these words, "Lord, if you had been here, my brother would not have died" (John 11:21). Intuitive, contemplative Mary came to Him next: "Lord, if you had been here, my brother would not have died" (v. 32). Both of the sisters were really saying, "If only . . . but You were too late!"

Martha and Mary had great faith in Jesus—so much that they were convinced He could have prevented Lazarus's death. They were upset with Jesus because He had not been prompt enough in responding to their needs.

From our perspective, Jesus is often late. By the time He arrives, bad things have happened to us, or we have messed up in some way. We have done too much of one thing or not enough of another. We have gone to excess in following the eccentricities of our minds, the wayward-ness of our inclinations, the lethargy of our wills, or the weakness of our constitutions. By the time we are aware of His presence, we haven't much in our hands to recommend us.

Jesus comes too late to prevent the wrongs people do to us, which we in turn pass on to others. He comes too late to stop war, disease, and sin. His tardiness angers us so that instead of admitting what we are—helpless, lost, crisis-prone, weak, and at best not wise enough, not loving enough—we are likely to excuse ourselves as victims who are not truly responsible.

Because of the kind of world we live in, Jesus will always seem to be too late to prevent wrong and ill, too late to stop us from our natural inclinations, too late to shelter us from the normal cycles of illness and death. God has given free choice, and sin and weakness are the results.

Sometimes Jesus is late deliberately, as He was when Lazarus died, so we might grow, be refined, and develop into strong people of God. We don't like that. We want life on our terms in our time frame. We want Jesus to be on time—so did Martha and Mary.[1]

I imagine the disciples wished they had left for Bethany earlier. Jesus had told them that Lazarus would be all right, but he wasn't; he was dead. When they encountered the mourners at the tomb, how could they explain these seeming contradictions? What excuses could they think of to cover for Jesus' seeming lack of concern?

I think Jesus was trying to teach them about God's timing, which often is very different from the way we tell time. He wanted Martha, Mary, and the disciples to learn to trust His timing and His love.

Waiting for Healing

The story of Lazarus reminds me of clinical situations in which it was very difficult for my patients to trust God's timing. Betty and Don had been married for nine years and were now in their early thirties. They had delayed starting a family until they completed their education and were established financially, but then it took two years of trying before Betty conceived.

When they first discovered Betty was pregnant, they told me they prayed daily for this baby. But as time went on, they began to refer more and more to what they had accomplished and how their plans were coming to fulfillment. I saw a subtle shift from dependence on God to reliance on themselves.

During an uneventful pregnancy, Betty gained a normal amount of weight, experienced routine aches and discomforts, and had the usual amount of swelling in her extremities. She was not very tall, but Don was over six feet and weighed 220 pounds. The baby took after his dad, and I estimated a fetal weight of nine pounds.

Shortly after her due date, Betty went into labor and progressed nicely in the active phase with Don present to offer encouragement and act as her coach. After more than eight hours of labor, Betty was completely dilated and ready to push. After two hours, the baby's head was crowning. As the head eased out, every obstetrician's nightmare happened. The head seemed to move back up into the birth canal, and the shoulders wouldn't come out—an event called shoulder dystocia.

We quickly flexed Betty's knees back onto her chest, asked her to push hard, and applied pressure just above her pubic bone to help the infant's shoulders dip below the pubic arch. With Betty and two nurses pushing, I was able to manipulate the baby beneath the pubic bone and out the birth canal.

The baby was stressed by the traumatic birth. His Apgar scores[2] at one and five minutes were low, and he required assistance to breathe properly. We transferred him to the intensive care unit, where he was finally stabilized. Over the next two days, Betty and Don's infant son, Scott, struggled to regain normality. Possible infection, blood sugar difficulties, and retention of fluid in the lungs posed temporary setbacks.

The young parents were frightened and rightly concerned about their baby. In our conversations they repeatedly asked, "Why would God let this happen when we prayed and waited for this baby so long? How could He do this to us?"

I reassured them that God was not punishing them but was reaching out to them and their baby with His healing touch. However, I could not help but recall their quick move from what God had accomplished to what they had succeeded in doing in the conception of this child. While God does not reach down and zap us for our lack of faith, He does use circumstances to draw us into a closer walk with Himself.

I said, "Betty and Don, just as you prayed fervently for this little boy to be yours, you now need to pray for his healing and then release the outcome to God. It is not easy, but you must trust Him to do His work in His time."

Three days passed, and although baby Scott was stable, there were few signs of improvement. The parents, grandparents, and church family prayed earnestly for healing. On the fourth day of his life, little Scott turned the corner. By God's mighty healing power, and with marvelous neonatologists providing care, he showed steady daily improvement. After a week, he was released from the neonatal intensive care unit. Today he is a healthy little boy.

Did God withhold His healing touch from Scott for three days? No. God was involved in Scott's healing all along, but He used that time to deal with Betty and Don in a powerful way. They were made aware of their dependence on God and their need to give Him the glory for all He enables them to accomplish—including conception. Their lives were changed, and they are now being used in their local church in a marvelous way as instruments of God's life-changing power.

Accepting Unanswered Prayer

As difficult as it may be, we need to trust the timing of healing to the One who is in charge of the process. From the raising of a man from a tomb to the raising of a baby from an isolette, God heals in His way and His time.

Sometimes the story doesn't end wonderfully. There are times when it seems the answer to prayer never comes. Such was the case for David Seamands, pastor, author, and friend of our family for as long as I can remember. In his book *If Only*, he tells of a heart-wrenching experience he and his wife, Helen, had in 1948, when they were young missionaries in India.

> Everything happened so quickly it left us shocked and numb. Our first son, healthy, ten-month-old David, had been cut down by fulminant bacilliary dysentery in a matter of hours. We were told later that fulminant meant "to strike like lightning," and that certainly was accurate. We buried him in the reddish soil of Bidar the next morning. Sympathetic crowds of dear Indian friends and fellow missionaries streamed through our home for a couple of days. My parents and brother (also missionaries) were with us too.
>
> But, after a few days, we were all alone. Night came, and our three-year-old daughter, dazed and disturbed by the disappearance of her little brother, had finally gone to sleep. The empty silence was deadening. The single hurricane lantern cast eerie shadows on the walls and twenty-foot ceilings of the old mission bungalow. Helen was playing the piano and we began to sing one of our favorite hymns, "Spirit of God, Descend Upon My Heart." We did fine until the words of the fourth stanza seemed to jump out and gnaw at something deep within us.
>
> > Teach me to feel that Thou art always nigh;
> > Teach me the struggles of the soul to bear.
> > To check the rising doubt, the rebel sigh,
> > Teach me the patience of unanswered prayer.
>
> All at once my voice broke and I began to fight back the tears. Unwanted and unwelcome thoughts which I had

pushed down suddenly erupted within me. Like molten lava, they spilled out into a bitter dialogue with God. "Lord, I don't understand. We left home and family and friends and came 10,000 miles to serve You as missionaries in India. We love You and we believe that You love us. Why did this happen? How could You have let this happen to us? Why? Why?"

In the coming days, God had to teach both of us more about life and death, love and suffering. . . . A devout British missionary friend once said to me, "You know, at times like these, in some ways it would be easier if we were atheists, wouldn't it?" At first I was shocked, but then I realized he was right. For it's the very fact of knowing God personally, and knowing that He not only exists but also loves us, which makes the difficulty even greater. Certainly we believe that ultimately God will be a part of the solution; but in the beginning, He seems a part of the problem. For the contradiction is more than rational; it is relational. Now it's not so much a philosophical question as it is a family quarrel![3]

As the saintly Teresa of Avila was one day "protesting to God the seemingly unjust suffering of a good person, she claimed God said to her, 'That's how I treat all My friends.' To which she replied, 'Well, Lord, now I understand why You have so few of them!'"[4]

Delayed Answers

So often when we have a need, we plead our case before God and nothing seems to happen. "Where is the answer?" we cry out. "Don't You even hear me when I pray? Don't You care? Your Word says that whatever I ask for in Your name will be done, and yet there has been no response to my plea." Instead of love or gratitude, we feel anger and resentment, as though we have been deceived.

I'm sure Martha and Mary must have had those feelings
even as they rushed out to meet Jesus. It is so hard to trust
God on His timetable and not ours.

Sylvia and Brad are dear friends who live in devotion to
God. They have raised their children in the faith, serve in
their local church, and are prayer warriors. When their nine-
teen-year-old daughter, Sarah, became ill with a chronic
kidney disease, her condition worsened dramatically. Her
name was placed on our church prayer chain, and people
across the country began praying for her recovery.

Sylvia and Brad trusted God for Sarah's complete recovery even as one kidney and then half of the other shut
down. Sarah had to begin renal dialysis three times a week
and grew progressively weaker. No one could understand
why God wasn't intervening in the life of this precious girl.

Days and weeks went by as Sarah continued in dialysis. When there was no improvement, her physicians
decided she would need a kidney transplant. A family
member was found to be a compatible donor, and surgery
was scheduled. As the day of the operation approached,
Sarah suddenly developed an upper respiratory infection,
and her doctors postponed the surgery until she recovered
from the virus.

To everyone's surprise, when Sarah improved, blood
tests showed that the one functioning kidney had improved. Two weeks later there was even more improvement, and the transplant was canceled. Some time later
Sarah was taken off dialysis.

Why did God delay in answering our prayers for Sarah?
Why did God allow this family to go through agonizing
emotions and grief when they had prayed and trusted so
completely? Why does He allow any of us to go through
the agony of praying, trusting, and hoping and then feeling intense disappointment when our prayers seem not

to be answered? These questions cannot be resolved on this side of eternity, but we do know that God does answer in His time and in His way. We are asked to trust His love and His timing.

We can learn from the spiritual truth Jesus revealed to the sisters and friends at Bethany. When He met a grieving Martha on the road and she reproached Him for not coming sooner, Jesus shared with her one of His most amazing statements, "I am the resurrection and the life. He who believes in me will live, even though he dies; and whoever lives and believes in me will never die. Do you believe this?" (John 11:25–26).

The religious teachers of Jesus' time would never have shared such profound truth with a woman. They wouldn't even talk to women in public places. Yet in this time of grief as well as in other instances during His ministry, Jesus opened His heart to speak some of His most important words to women. He took them seriously and knew they were just as able—and perhaps more open at times—as the men to receive words of truth.

Jesus was deeply moved by the grief of Martha, Mary, and their friends, and He wept. He entered into their grief, and His compassion was proof to those looking on, not of His power but of His love.

The moment of truth came when Jesus asked the bystanders to roll away the stone from Lazarus's tomb. Martha protested, "Lord, he has been dead four days—it will smell terrible!" They were talking about smells when He was thinking about resurrection.

Jesus said to her, "Did I not tell you that if you believed, you would see the glory of God?" (John 11:40). There it is—believe first and then see. God's timing is so different from ours. We want to see and then we'll believe.

Even after the stone was rolled away, Jesus delayed again, this time to pray. But to Him prayer wasn't delay. It was part of the process, as it should be with us, con-

stantly talking with the Father and seeking His will. We
need to employ prayer and Scripture to defeat Satan.

Then, finally, Jesus said, "Lazarus, come out!" (John
11:43). And Lazarus did.

Why all the delay? Why take so long—at Bethany, in
Lexington, Kentucky, or in Portland, Chicago, or Boston?

Why did Jesus take time for loving words of encouragement with Mary and Martha? Why did He weep with
them and their friends? Because He is loving and compassionate, supportive and sympathetic, our friend as well
as our Savior, our shepherd as well as our master.

God does the same for us today, and then in His time
and way, we begin to see the glory of God. Not because
everything turns out just as we wanted it to, but because
the God of glory is with us and in us and is infusing every
circumstance of our lives with His glory, love, and eternal
healing.

eight

Restoration for Our Children

*J*esus and His disciples were on their way to Nain, a village about six miles from Nazareth. As so often happened, they were not alone on the road but were accompanied by crowds of people seeking a miracle or hoping to see one. As they approached the town gate of Nain, they saw a funeral procession of a young man, the only son of a widow.

As Jesus watched the procession, His heart went out to the grieving mother, and He said to her, "Don't cry." Then He walked over to the coffin and touched it. The procession stopped, and the people looked at Jesus, waiting to see what He would do (Luke 7:11–13).

Interrupting a funeral was probably as socially unacceptable then as it is now. What the crowd didn't realize was that Jesus had another perspective on death—and life. In telling the grieving mother, "Don't cry," He was not forbidding her to weep for her loss. Rather, He was encouraging her not to mourn any longer because there

105

was truly life after death and—in this case—restoration now.

As He touched the bier, Jesus said to the deceased, "'Young man, I say to you, get up!' The dead man sat up and began to talk, and Jesus gave him back to his mother" (Luke 7:14–15). Can you imagine the astonishment of the mourners? Those who had planned to spend their day in sadness and mourning were now filled with awe and fear, and they began to glorify God. "'A great prophet has appeared among us,' they said. 'God has come to help his people'" (Luke 7:16).

In this story Jesus moved quickly to restore the dead young man to his mother. While we don't know if tears fell from His eyes, we do know He was moved with compassion. In the resurrection of Lazarus (see chapter 7), Jesus was so moved by the sadness and loss His friends felt that He wept with them. Jesus, truly God and truly man, entered fully into human life then and continues to now. As the writer of the book of Hebrews tells us, "We do not have a high priest who is unable to sympathize with our weaknesses, but we have one who has been tempted in every way, just as we are—yet was without sin. Let us then approach the throne of grace with confidence, so that we may receive mercy and find grace to help us in our time of need" (Heb. 4:15–16).

We don't often think of a funeral as a place for healing to take place, and yet it can be. Everyone affected by the death of a loved one needs some kind of healing, and the mother and friends of the young man experienced it that day in Nain in a miraculous way.

More Than a Resurrection

This story is not only about the resurrection of a young man from the grip of death. It is also one of the many

statements Jesus made about the status of women and the
legalistic rituals of the Jewish people. In His words and
actions, Jesus was saying, "I care. I understand. I came to
restore you and to give each of you life. I came to show
you how much your heavenly Father cares about you and
how He wants to bless you so that your life can be a blessing to others."

If we had been there that day, we would have seen the
corpse, which had been lovingly prepared for burial just
hours after the death, since interment would take place
within the first day. From various Bible passages, we can
see the sequence of preparation.

"As soon as the individual expired, the eldest son or
nearest relative present would close the eyes of the
deceased (Gen. 46:4). . . . The mouth was bound shut
(John 11:44), the body washed (Acts 9:37) and then
anointed with aromatic ointments (John 12:7; 19:39;
Mark 16:1; Luke 24:1). The body was then wrapped in
cloth (usually linen, Matt. 27:59; John 11:44), although
individuals of high rank would frequently be clothed in
fine garments."[1]

Burial followed as soon as possible after a death, no
doubt because of sanitary reasons (Acts 5:6, 10; 8:1–2).
However, sometimes there could be a delay (Acts
9:37–39). The Gospels' details about the preparation for
the burial of our Lord—the ointment and spices (Matt.
26:12; Luke 23:56) and the mixture of myrrh and aloes—
are confirmed in records of rabbis of that time. At times
the cost of funerals was so excessive that it caused serious difficulties to the poor, since they did not want to be
outdone by their neighbors in showing respect for their
dead.[2]

In the case of this young man, the mother would have
been the one to close his eyes and then seek the help of
her neighbors and friends in preparing his body. After it
was wrapped in linens, they placed the body on a bier or

open casket, which was carried by friends, servants, or relatives. "The procession was led by professional mourners,
followed by family members who filled the air with cries
of sadness and agony."[3]

The Jews believed that children benefited or suffered
according to the spiritual state of their parents. Therefore, this woman would have had double anguish: She
not only lost her son but also had to bear the burden of
feeling she had contributed to his suffering and death.
Sickness was regarded as punishment for sin as well as
an atonement for wrongdoing. Someone who died under
fifty years of age was said to be "cut off" from God. One
who died suddenly was said to have been "swallowed up";
death after one day's illness was a "rejection"; after two
days it was "despair"; after four days a "reproof"; and
after five days a "natural death." The manner of death
was considered a good or bad omen bearing on the person's future in eternity.[4]

The ancient tradition was that since women brought
death into the world, they should also lead the way in the
funeral procession. The grieving mother would have
walked alone followed by the paid mourners.[5]

Throughout Jesus' ministry, He seemed intent on rec-
ognizing the proper place of women in His kingdom,
regardless of their present circumstances. For Him to move
toward the mother was a break from tradition, which
insisted that a man not talk with a woman in public, and
especially not a stranger.[6] He would have known the criticism that would come His way from the religious leaders, but He did not hesitate.

Yes, surely God visited His people that day. Unrestricted
by tradition, Jesus moved through the barriers of polite-
ness and the laws about uncleanness and brought life.
Clean and unclean were meaningless categories to the
One who holds the power to heal and restore.

A Baby Restored to Life

The story of the widow of Nain reminds me of a woman whose child was near death's door. Although this child was not dead, Jesus' spiritual presence was just as real to her mother as was His physical presence at Nain.

Early in her second pregnancy, Frances came to my office for obstetrical care. Her first delivery had been uneventful, and she didn't expect a problem this time. However, in the twentieth week of the pregnancy, two traumatic events occurred.

First, a routine ultrasound scan confirmed that the female infant had a significant abnormality. The diaphragm, which is supposed to separate the abdominal and chest cavities, was everted into the chest, allowing the stomach to press against the lungs and restrict their capacity to expand. This condition, *diaphragmatic hernia,* can prevent the lungs from developing fully. This is not life threatening while the baby is inside the uterus, because the baby receives oxygen from the mother's blood via the placenta and the umbilical cord. When the child is born, however, if the lungs are compressed or have not fully developed, the baby will be unable to breathe on its own. Frances was devastated by this news.

The second traumatic event was that Frances's husband chose this time to leave her. Without even a good-bye, he wrote a brief note telling her that he did not love her anymore and had met another woman he wanted to be with.

I continue to be amazed at how frequently infidelity occurs during a pregnancy. Expectant fathers should show gentle care, loving concern, and supportive assistance throughout the pregnancy. Yet there is something in certain men that allows them to impregnate a woman and then remove themselves emotionally from the situation, finding the pregnant body repulsive rather than finding joy in the very life they have helped to create.

Frances was strong, but with no husband to rely on for emotional support during the last difficult days of the pregnancy, I feared she might not survive psychologically. Her family was furious with her husband, but they rallied around her with encouragement and prayers, wisely directing all their counsel toward preparing for the birth of the child.

I told Frances that we would watch her baby very carefully and try to bring her to a mature gestational age before we had to deliver her. If we found that the lungs were becoming too compromised, we would have to deliver her prematurely. I encouraged Frances to pray diligently that the baby would be able to stay in the womb close to term (forty weeks). I also arranged for her to begin seeing a marriage counselor and a psychologist to help her deal with the stress she was facing.

In the weeks that followed, Frances felt abandoned, but she tried to adjust to being alone with her toddler while dealing with a difficult pregnancy. Her baby grew slowly, but the lungs continued to develop. I encouraged Frances that we might be able to reach thirty-seven weeks gestation before inducing labor.

As the time drew near, I notified the pediatrician, the neonatologist, and the pediatric surgeons, so that we would have a plan of action for the postdelivery period. When week thirty-seven came, I scheduled Frances for induction of labor. Because she had not heard from her husband, her sister was to be her labor coach. Although they were excited about the arrival of the baby, they felt a cloud of sorrow over the birth defect and the absence of Frances's husband.

The induction of labor went well, and as Frances had regular contractions, the baby's heart rate remained strong. After a few hours, Frances was completely dilated and began pushing. Suddenly, the baby's heart rate dropped from 150 to 75 and did not increase in spite of all our efforts to correct it. Rapidly we prepared this very frightened young woman for a forceps delivery, called in all the other specialists, and arranged for a room in the operating suite to be cleared for the inevitable surgery the baby would need.

The forceps delivery went quite easily, and as I suctioned the baby's mouth and nose and handed the fragile body to the neonatologist, I silently prayed. She quickly placed a tube in the baby's airway and attempted to ventilate her lungs. "I can barely move any air into her lungs," she said. As often happens in these situations, events transpired in rapid succession with orders being called out, nurses running in all directions to find needed medication and equipment, and physicians working to restore the basic functions of life. The silent infant was quickly shifted to a neonatal transporter to move her to the operating room.

It was the procession of doctors, nurses, and aides following the rolling isolette with the pale baby girl inside and the sobs of Frances and her sister echoing through the delivery room that suddenly drew my mind to the story of the widow of Nain. It seemed as if this baby were being carried on a bier and that Frances, now alone without her husband, was leading a funeral procession. I spoke the only words I could muster, "Frances, she is going to make it. Don't cry, just pray." My words belied my own lack of faith that this child would be raised from her bier alive.

As soon as the baby was anesthetized, the surgeon opened her chest, decompressed it by pushing the abdominal contents down, and secured a mesh graft in the place where the original diaphragm should have been in order to hold the stomach in place. The right lung and a portion of the left were salvageable, and soon the anesthesiologist was able to ventilate the baby adequately and her color improved. Her heart rate returned to normal more slowly, but at least she was alive and improving.

Following the operation, baby Janice progressed well, and Frances was able to hold her that evening and to begin nursing her the next day. She was a tough little girl, and she fought back from the insult of surgery to make a good recovery.

When Janice was three months old, Frances brought her to my office. As I held her little angel in my arms, I said, "Frances, God has touched her twice. He created her, and then He reached out to heal her when her lifeless body was wheeled out of the delivery room. He is speaking to you and telling you that He loves you and will care for you always."

As we looked at each other, we both began to cry, and then we hugged. The mother from Nain had her child back. Janice has continued to develop normally, and you would never know that she had been critically ill. Today she is energetic, bright, and charming. More importantly, her mother often tells her how God spared her life because He has something important for her to do. Frances also takes every opportunity to witness to others about the miracle of restoration in her daughter's life.

"Don't Be Afraid"

Another child restored to life by Jesus was the twelve-year-old daughter of Jairus, a ruler of the synagogue. As Jairus came with his urgent plea, he found himself in the middle of a crowd welcoming Jesus back to Galilee (Luke 8:40–42). He was also made painfully aware that he was not the only one seeking Jesus' attention as "the crowds almost crushed him" (v. 42).

As they were walking toward Jairus's home, a woman with a hemorrhage touched Jesus, causing a distraction that stopped their progress (see chapter 4). Jairus wanted Jesus to hurry along to heal his daughter, not to be detained by someone He couldn't even locate. Yet Jesus took the time to find the woman who had been healed. As He was talking with her, a messenger came from Jairus's home to tell him, "Your daughter is dead. Don't bother the teacher any more" (Luke 8:49). When Jesus heard this, He looked at the suffering father and said, "Don't be afraid; just believe, and she will be healed" (Luke 8:50).

Just as Jesus delayed until Lazarus was already buried, so He delayed in this instance, waiting until Jairus's daughter was dead. The loving father could not understand the delay any more than Martha and Mary could. But the Lord has His own timing, then and now. He was really asking Jairus to trust His timetable for the healing.

As we have seen several times already, reliance on God's timing appears to be essential to complete healing and well-being. Yet it is so difficult to be patient when one you love is dying before your eyes. Of course, this does not mean that we should delay medical treatment when it is needed, but it does mean that if we do not see healing when we want it to happen, we should continue to trust the Lord.

When they arrived at Jairus's home, Jesus took Peter, James, John, and the child's parents in with Him. As was the custom, relatives and friends were wailing with grief for the dead child. Jesus told them, "Stop wailing. She is not dead but asleep" (Luke 8:52). Even through their grief, this was so preposterous that they laughed at Him. They knew she was dead.

Jesus took the child by the hand and said, "My child, get up!" (v. 53). When she heard that, even in death, "her spirit returned, and at once she stood up" (v. 55). Of course Jairus and his wife were astonished and might have expected a remarkable request from Jesus, but He told them only to give their daughter something to eat. Her miraculous healing did not take away her need for the basic necessities of life. Jesus knew that she needed food and water. In the same way, we need to seek the things that are necessary to sustain us physically, even when we pray for divine healing.

It may have seemed strange to them that Jesus asked them not to tell anyone what had happened (v. 56). In any case, it was impossible for others not to know, since family and friends were already gathered around the house.

Jesus clearly saw a finer line between life and death than we do, and that fine line is one we can hold to when someone we love dies. Someday, in an instant, that one and all who die in the Lord will be brought back together, and we will know them in joyous reunion.

Angels in the Pool

I know the feeling of absolute panic when a child is near death. When our oldest son, Philip, was three years old, we were vacationing in Florida at the home of friends. After a delicious meal, my friend Steve and I decided to go out by the pool to talk. Philip wanted to come along, so I put a life jacket on him but told him he could not go in the water because he had just eaten.

Deep in conversation, Steve and I did not see Philip take off his life jacket and wade into the shallow end of the pool. Then Steve suddenly asked, "Where is Phil?" We glanced about the deck and didn't see him. At that moment we both saw an object on the bottom of the shallow end of the pool. Steve dove into the water and literally threw Philip to me on the side. I caught his limp body and began resuscitation efforts while pleading with God to save his life. There is no feeling worse than trying to resuscitate your own child. I breathed into him and pumped his little heart. After what seemed an eternity, he began to cough and move. He then spit up a large quantity of water and weakly asked, "What happened?"

I clutched him to me and answered, "You're okay. You just swallowed a little water."

"Thank You, God," I said aloud. "Thank You!" My son who was dead was now alive again. Many years later, Philip told us that he saw angels while he was on the bottom of the pool, and I am convinced they directed our attention to him before it was too late.

I understood that day how Jairus must have felt when he was trying to get Jesus to come with him to heal his daughter. There is no plea as desperate as that of a parent whose child is dying. We think of the parents around the world who are pleading for the lives of their children. It must break God's heart to see His little ones suffering so, for they are the ones to whom the kingdom of God belongs (Mark 10:14). As Jesus took a child in His arms, He said to the disciples, "Whoever welcomes one of these little children in my name welcomes me; and whoever welcomes me does not welcome me but the one who sent me" (Mark 9:37). We must be attentive to the physical, emotional, and spiritual needs of all children, not only our own. Their future and ours depend on this.

Worse Than Death

The stories of the widow of Nain, Jairus's daughter, Janice, and Philip, as well as many other near-death experiences are emotionally wrenching. However, there is another kind of near-death experience that may seem even worse. When an adolescent or grown child becomes involved in a destructive or criminal way of life, a parent sometimes feels it would be easier if the child had died. When the aberrant behavior continues for months and even years, the toll this takes on parents is often harder than a death.

Tammie was my patient, and she and her husband, Ben, had become personal friends. They were dedicated Christians who seemed to have a wonderful relationship with their children; they had spent time with them in many activities and had raised them in the church. I was shocked, therefore, when Tammie came in for an appointment and responded to my inquiry about the children by becoming tearful and silent for several minutes.

"Tammie, I'm sorry—it looks as if I touched a very tender subject."

"Yes, David, you did," she replied almost apologetically. "It's really a long story. Could I call you at home and talk to you and Linda about it?"

"Certainly. Any time you feel like it, just give us a call."

A couple of weeks later Tammie telephoned. "I'm sorry it took me so long to get back to you, but it is so embarrassing that I just didn't have the nerve to call right away. Billy isn't at home anymore."

Billy was just sixteen years old, so I knew he wasn't away at college. Since it was the middle of the school year, he wouldn't be on vacation. Billy was a handsome, quiet, and bright young man who had always been very popular with his peers, did well in school, and played baseball. Also, he had always attended youth group as well as the worship services at church. I couldn't imagine what Tammie was saying about Billy.

I could sense the tears welling up as Tammie continued. "We first began to notice something was wrong when the principal called to tell us that Billy had been skipping school. His grades had not been as good in the last semester, but we felt it was because he was taking a heavier load of classes. I had noticed that he was locking the door to his room more often and listening to louder music, but I thought this was probably normal for a boy his age. He also seemed to need a lot more sleep; his eyes were often red and tired, and he didn't take the same pride in his appearance as he had.

"We had always done things together as a family, but now Billy didn't have time for us anymore. The kids he used to run around with were no longer at our house, and Billy went out more. We felt that we needed to give him his space, so we didn't say very much. When we did ask where he was going and who he was going to see, we received increasingly vague answers. Ben and Billy had always been so close, and it was hard on Ben to see him pull away like that, but we assumed it was normal adolescent behavior.

"Then Billy was arrested for driving under the influence of alcohol, and we had to go to the city detention center to bail him out. When we asked him what had happened, his only response was sullen anger. Ben told him he was grounded and couldn't drive the car for a month. Billy blew a fuse and ran out of the house. Ben went after him in the car and was able to bring him back home that night, but it was just the beginning of more fights and less communication. We sought counseling from a trusted friend, but Billy would not answer any of the questions. At one session, there was discussion about putting Billy in a facility for juvenile alcoholics, to which he screamed that he was not an alcoholic and would not go. Ben and I felt as if we were going crazy—we didn't know what to do.

"One night Billy left the house without permission to attend a party on a nearby farm. A fight occurred, and some kids were arrested, including Billy. This time he had to stay in jail in spite of our protests. There was a court hearing because one of the boys in the fight had been seriously injured, and his parents sued five sets of parents for damages. Billy insisted that another kid had started it, but this didn't really matter because by now he was in serious trouble. We later found out that he had been doing drugs for months and was addicted to crack cocaine as well as being an alcoholic. Now we wonder how we could not have suspected what was wrong, how we could have been so blind."

"Tammie, I'm so sorry," I responded. "But you shouldn't blame yourself, because many other parents have been fooled by children who have become addicts. The telltale signs are not always obvious, and parents often write them off as 'being a kid'—just as you and Ben did. What matters now is that you need to help Billy get his life back. This will probably require some changes in your relationship with him so that healing can occur. If you spend all your time feeling guilty and sorry for yourself, you won't be able to help him when he returns home and needs you both."

Billy was placed in a rehabilitation center in another state where he dried out and received quality counseling about the issues in his life. As Tammie and Ben thought about their relationship with him, they realized they had not spent the time they should have in quality conversation to stay current with him in his teen years. The telltale signs were there, but they didn't recognize them.

It takes tough love to rear a child today. We parents want our children to like us, but sometimes we won't be well liked by our children when we have to make decisions about their way of life that are contrary to what they want. We have to remember that we did not become parents to win a popularity contest. Our job is to prepare our children to be responsible citizens as well as followers of Christ. We need to set an example of consistent living. Young people can see right through hypocrisy and inconsistency and may react against adults who behave this way by choosing an antisocial lifestyle. As Jesus told His disciples, we are not to hinder children from coming to Him; however, we are to hinder them from going toward Satan and evil ways.

In his book *Life on the Edge,* James Dobson says that this generation has been bombarded with more antifamily rhetoric than any other before it. Messages about drugs, sex, and violence are constantly before young people today.[7]

In spite of parents who loved him and did their best to expose him to religious training and provide a nurturing family, Billy got in with the wrong crowd and still has not recovered. After his time at the rehabilitation center, he returned home and began using drugs again. He was arrested for driving without a license and also for violation of probation.

Tammie and Ben feel that they are living in a hell on earth. I have talked with them often, trying to help them see that they did the best they could at the time. "You cannot continue blaming yourselves. All you can do now is to love Billy and pray for him."

Tammie has been surrounded by loving friends who have prayed with her and encouraged her. Her sorrow and the fellowship of Christians has brought her into a deeper relationship with Christ. I told her the story of the widow of Nain and asked her to visualize Billy lying on a funeral bier in a lifeless state. Next I encouraged her to see Jesus coming over to Billy and touching him, giving renewed life in resurrection power. Then we prayed for Billy and also for Tammie and Ben, that healing would occur in their family. She feels assured that God will touch him and restore him to his family, healthy and whole.

No matter what your sorrow, no matter how severe or devastating it may be, Jesus stands ready and willing to touch the bier of sorrow in your life and bring healing and restoration. We all hope the tragedies of life will pass us by, but when they come too close, we need to avail ourselves of the resources we have in Jesus Christ and from His people. These can help to mend even the most painful grief or damaged relationship. Won't you let Him dry your tears?

~~~~~~~~~~~~~~~~~~~~~~~~~~~~

nine

Jesus Cares for Senior Citizens

*t*wo of Jesus' healing miracles touched the lives of women we would call senior citizens. The first of these was a woman who had suffered from a crippling disease for eighteen years. If anyone had a reason not to get to church, she did. Doctor Luke tells us that "she was bent over and could not straighten up at all" (Luke 13:11).

Think of some of the excuses you have heard—or used—for not attending church:

"It's cold."
"It's raining."
"I'm not feeling well."
"I'm tired."
"I just couldn't get everyone dressed."
"I have to get this work done."

This woman could have said, "I just can't make it. My legs and back are killing me."

We have all seen people like this woman trying to nego-
tiate the simplest tasks, and they are painful to watch.
She, however, seemed intent on staying connected with
the people of God, no matter how she felt. On the Sabbath
she was in the synagogue where Jesus was to teach. In the
middle of His message, He noticed her crippled condition.
Jesus reacted sympathetically, as we would, but He reached
out to her as only God can. He singled her out, asking her
not merely to look at Him or even to stand, but to make
her way to the front of the synagogue.

Was it necessary to make a spectacle of her in order to
heal her? Could she not have received healing where she
sat, bent over? Jesus could have gone to her, or He could
have healed her at home. Yet there was significance in her
being in the place of worship, as difficult as it was to get
there. She went to the place where God was known to be
at work and joined Him there. In spite of her years of suffering, she trusted God to satisfy all of her needs, and she
wanted to show Him her love.

The crippled woman's presence also said that she was
seeking from God more than she could ever receive from
anyone else. No doctors had been able to help her, and
while she probably had given up hope of being healed,
she still sought spiritual consolation. This woman clearly
had a desire for God's presence in her life.

When she arrived at the front, Jesus spoke to her,
"'Woman, you are set free from your infirmity.' Then he
put his hands on her, and immediately she straightened
up and praised God" (Luke 13:12–13).

Can you imagine the electricity that must have gone
through her body when the Master touched her and those
old bones and joints, which had been crooked and
inflamed for years, were suddenly able to move normally?
Because Jesus had asked her to come to Him, she was now
able to look directly into the face of the Great Physician.
No longer stooped over with pain, she could see His eyes

as she thanked Him for caring enough about an elderly woman to stop His teaching and heal her body.

However, there were other faces she could see as well—some probably compassionate, some inquisitive, some irritated that the teaching had been interrupted. As she turned, one face she saw was that of the ruler of the synagogue as he indignantly declared, "There are six days for work. So come and be healed on those days, not on the Sabbath" (Luke 13:14).

Have you ever felt excited about an event or been touched in your spirit by a blessing only to have someone demean what you have just experienced? This woman was overjoyed by the possibility of living pain-free for the rest of her life, and now she heard her minister rebuke her for receiving a miracle on the wrong day of the week!

This reaction seemed to be just what Jesus was waiting for. He answered, "You hypocrites! Doesn't each of you on the Sabbath untie his ox or donkey from the stall and lead it out to give it water? Then should not this woman, a daughter of Abraham, whom Satan has kept bound for eighteen long years, be set free on the Sabbath day from what bound her?" (Luke 13:15–16).

Jesus was not attributing this woman's malady to sin; rather, He was indicating that Satan had used his power to keep this woman in bondage to her disease. I take this to mean that we need to rebuke Satan whenever we see someone in the grasp of a chronic disease. This woman was a dedicated churchgoer, and yet Jesus knew that Satan was trying to bind and defeat her.

Losses That Bind Older Women

You probably know some older people who have become more and more isolated from others, and often with less excuse than this crippled woman. A major reason is the presence of disease that binds and cripples. The woman in Luke 13 may have suffered from the degenerative process of osteoporosis, which causes weak spots to develop in bones so they do not support the body well and are susceptible to fractures. You may have seen older women today who are bent over, sometimes almost double, and can barely move because of the bone breakdown associated with osteoporosis. Exercise and calcium are important preventatives, but if estrogen is not present, the calcium will not remain in the bones, and they will become weak.

Today we can prescribe estrogen to menopausal women to help keep their bones strong. Not only does estrogen bind calcium to the bones, it also significantly decreases the incidence of heart attack, improves the condition of the skin, decreases the risk of Alzheimer's disease, and improves memory. It may also decrease the risk of colon cancer and improve vision.[1]

I see older women in my practice almost every day. While some of them are very involved in church and in doing good for others, some use their age as an excuse not to be involved. They have time to go out to lunch with their friends or shop but not to take part in spiritual activities. This is a shame, because they have so much to offer from a lifetime of learning and experience. I sometimes think these women are also bound, just as was the crippled woman in Jesus' time. Their negative attitudes keep them disconnected from involvements that would be of great benefit to them. Some of the factors that keep older people from experiencing the fullness of God in their lives are:

loneliness
anger
bitterness
poor health

loss of self-esteem
financial difficulties
emotional problems
negative behaviors

These factors interact with each other and often weave a web that leaves many older people feeling disenfranchised and isolated from others.

We have a responsibility to aid senior citizens and help them cope with the problems of age. Jesus was acutely aware of this and brought healing and comfort to the elderly as well as to younger adults. On the Sabbath when He healed the crippled woman, He delighted most of the people and enraged the religious authorities. Every time He reached out to women in compassion, He further kindled the anger of the establishment. Jesus knew what He was doing and what He was facing. As He gave Himself to and for women, He was giving Himself for all of us.

Healed to Serve

Mark 1:21–34 tells us about another Sabbath when Jesus taught and healed in the synagogue. When He was finished, He went with James and John to the home of Simon and Andrew. There they found that Simon Peter's mother-in-law was in bed with a fever (vv. 29–31). This must not have been merely a low-grade fever, or she would not have been in bed.

When Jesus heard she was sick, He went in to her, took her by the hand, and helped her up. Immediately the fever left her, she felt well, and she began to serve them all.

Matthew (8:14–15) and Luke (4:38–39) also tell this story with a slightly different emphasis. In Luke, when Jesus leans over and rebukes the fever, He confronts the illness as He would an evil spirit. To *rebuke* means to admonish, remonstrate, punish. Jesus was admonishing the fever to come out of her so that she could be the woman she was intended to be.

Remember, this was the Sabbath. Jesus had just healed a man in the synagogue, and now in the home of Peter He was again rejecting the belief that persons should not be healed on the day of rest. He was also making a statement that women deserve healing as much as men. This time there was no one to criticize the Great Physician for His act of compassion.

Mark's Gospel says that Jesus raised her up. I have wondered if this might be a reference to resurrection, when we will all be raised up from the diseases of life and death to spiritual health in the presence of God.

If we use a bit of imagination as we read Mark 1:31, we can see Simon Peter's mother-in-law serving the family and friends. Then as we read the next verses, we can well believe that she had a very busy day. "That evening after sunset the people brought to Jesus all the sick and demon-possessed. The whole town gathered at the door, and Jesus healed many who had various diseases" (Mark 1:32–34).

I believe this story records one of the most significant healings of Jesus, but not for the reasons we have already mentioned. Not because she was a woman, and not because it happened on the Sabbath. I see great importance in what Simon Peter's mother-in-law did after she was healed. She could have arisen from her sick bed and been served, but the Gospel writers tell us that she served Jesus and the others. In His interactions with women, Jesus told them to do something: "Go and sin no more; go and tell others; come to the front. . . ." In this instance, she got up and on her own began to serve.

Isn't that why we are healed? We are made whole physically so that we can be about God's business—serving others. Rising from a sick bed to serve a meal may not sound all that significant, but that is the work she had to do. That was her role of service.

The larger purpose of healing is not just that we will feel better physically and emotionally. It is so that our healing will bring glory to God, restoring our health so that our lives will serve His purposes and glorify His name. If we are healed, it is so that we can return to what God is doing in the world and serve His purposes. It is wonderful to be healed, but it is more wonderful to be healed and then to begin to serve others. It is great to ponder the miraculous event and draw closer to God, but it is greater yet to invest the energy we receive in those who still need a healing touch. Remember, there is nothing saving in the world except self-sacrifice. The ultimate acts of "saving" are all self-sacrificial, from Jesus' death to our acts of intervention for others.

Serving in Spite of Pain

My mother died in 1995 after a long battle with cancer. She was diagnosed with cancer of the appendix seven years earlier at the age of seventy-six. She had surgery and then radiation therapy and chemotherapy. Her life expectancy at the time of her original diagnosis was only two years, and yet she lived seven. We had prayed for healing for her, and we believe our prayers were answered, because she lived five years longer than anyone thought she would.

In spite of the fact that my mother was receiving chemotherapy and radiation for much of the seven years she lived after her diagnosis, she continued to serve in her home, church, and community. She believed with all of her heart that God gave her those years to love and serve her family and the many other people who needed her touch. She visited sick persons and cheered them up, even when she did not feel well. She prepared meals for others on days when it would have been far easier to stay home and rest. She continued to be active in her church, to host functions in her home for women's groups from the church and community, and to sing in the choir. Also, she regularly invited the family over for Sunday dinner, and she supported my father in his retirement career as an administrator at Asbury College. Her insistence on staying connected with family, friends, church, and community was a great inspiration to all of us.

My mother believed that we are healed to serve. She also believed that healing is a continuum whereby we may be healed to varying degrees here, but that we will be made completely whole in our life with Christ in heaven.

Something More to Do

A story in the Book of Acts underscores the idea of our being restored so that we can serve. In the city of Joppa lived a woman known as Tabitha, or Dorcas, "who was always doing good and helping the poor" (Acts 9:36). Although we aren't told her age, she was probably advanced in years, because her subsequent illness and death were of great concern to the widows of the community. When Dorcas died, the Christians there called for Peter to come to them at once.

When he arrived, they took Peter to the room where Dorcas lay. "All the widows stood around him, crying and showing him the robes and other clothing that Dorcas had made while she was still with them" (Acts 9:39). After sending everyone out of the room, Peter knelt to pray. Then he stood and spoke to the dead woman, "Tabitha, get up" (v. 40). At this, she opened her eyes and sat up. As you can imagine, there was great rejoicing in the church. The implication was that Dorcas would continue to do her good works for the poor, just as she had before. God gives all of us life in order that we can serve Him and other people. God continues to be active in extending life for some whom He needs to accomplish His purposes. One such person was Patricia.

In 1986, Patricia was facing the sunset of her life, and she couldn't understand why the Lord didn't just take her home. She had lived a full life as a nurse and then as the first female hospital administrator in the United States, receiving a good deal of acclaim for her work. She was a tall, stately woman who had been active and even feisty wherever she went, but now she had cancer and finally had to be admitted to a nursing facility.

One March night when she was very sick, Patricia thought she saw Jesus waiting for her. When she woke up, she felt angry that she was still alive. She asked her pastor, "Why didn't the Lord just take me? What good am I to anyone now?" As he thought about this, her pastor told Patricia that he felt she had something more to do for God here on earth.

Patricia's birthday was on Sunday, March 17, and the youth group from her church decided to have a St. Patrick's Day party in her room to celebrate her birthday. As they ate and sang together, she told them about her life and how God had led her through many experiences. All of the young people were in tears as they felt the impact of her life.

Later that day, the nursing home called her pastor to say that Patricia was dying. He was not surprised—she had done her last work. He went to the nursing home and prayed with her, and within the hour Patricia was in the presence of the Lord she so much wanted to see.

What can the elderly do when they feel useless? Many feel that no one wants to listen to them, and yet we need their wisdom and experience to encourage us and help us avoid mistakes. Some senior citizens can visit the sick or prepare meals for those who are grieving or in need. They can call others on the phone even if they can't get out, or they can write cards and letters. They can do as my eighty-three-year-old father did when he finally retired yet another time—he volunteered in his community and church. Whatever your degree of strength and mobility, God has something for you to do before He takes you home.[2]

"At Even Ere the Sun Was Set"

There is a wonderful old hymn by Henry Twells about the day on which Jesus healed Peter's mother-in-law. It is one that has been used in churches to remind us of the healing presence of Christ with us today.

> At even ere the sun was set
> The sick, O Lord, around thee lay;
> O in what divers pains they met!
> O with what joy they went away!
>
> Once more 'tis eventide, and we
> Oppressed with various ills, draw near;
> What if thy form we cannot see?
> We know and feel that thou art here.
>
> O Saviour Christ, our woes dispel;
> For some are sick, and some are sad,
> And some have never loved thee well,
> And some have lost the love they had.
>
> O Saviour Christ, thou too art Man;
> Thou hast been troubled, tempted, tried;
> Thy kind but searching glance can scan
> The very wounds that shame would hide.

Thy touch has still its ancient power,
No word from thee can fruitless fall;
Hear in this solemn evening hour,
And in thy mercy heal us all.

There is always work to do in the kingdom, and age isn't very important in determining who will do it. There are sick people to be visited, poor people to be clothed, hungry people to be fed, lonely people to be comforted, prisoners to be encouraged, the homeless to be aided, and shut-ins to visit. With the welfare reforms happening in our country, it is going to be even more essential for the people of God to become involved in caring for those who are less fortunate.

God identifies Himself in special ways with those who are lonely, who feel rejected, who seem undesirable. In his prophecy, Isaiah wrote of the Messiah who would come not as a glorious king at first, but as one from whom we would turn our faces.

Who has believed our message
    and to whom has the arm of the Lord been revealed?
He grew up before him like a tender shoot,
    and like a root out of dry ground.
He had no beauty or majesty to attract us to him,
    nothing in his appearance that we should desire him.
He was despised and rejected by men,
    a man of sorrows, and familiar with suffering.
Like one from whom men hide their faces
    he was despised, and we esteemed him not.
Surely he took up our infirmities
    and carried our sorrows,
yet we considered him stricken by God,
    smitten by him, and afflicted.
But he was pierced for our transgressions,
    he was crushed for our iniquities;
the punishment that brought us peace was upon him,
    and by his wounds we are healed.

Isaiah 53:1–5

No matter what your age or physical condition, God does have something for you to do. Even if your body is shutting down physically, that doesn't mean you have to shut down mentally, emotionally, and spiritually.

My father-in-law, Thomas Carruth, had dementia in his latter years and required skilled nursing care. But as he sat in his chair near many others who had similar problems, he sang hymns or prayed out loud. It was all he could do, but it was apparently why God left him on this earth for his last few years. When we visited him, members of other families would tell us that Dr. Tom had led their relative to Christ in the nursing home. We couldn't understand it, but we knew that God chose to bless others through Dr. Tom's infirmity, making him a means through whom He could draw persons to Himself.

Yes, God does have something for you to do, no matter what your age may be.

ten

What Makes the Difference in a Woman's Health?

*i*f you have ever taken part in a survey by the health-care industry, you were asked about your family health history, any diseases you have had, medications you take, and your relationship with your physicians. The interviewer probably also asked you to rate your own health as excellent, good, fair, or poor. Since these researchers usually represent hospitals or medical insurance companies, their interest is only in your physical health. One curious result of such surveys is that some people whose medical history shows them to be at the peak of health may rate themselves only as *good* or *fair*, while others will follow a string of ailments with a rating of *excellent*.

I prefer to ask my patients questions that will integrate what I am finding out medically with what else is happening in their lives—considering the whole person. On any given day in my practice, it is not unusual for me to see two patients who have the same disease or disorder, perhaps an ovarian cyst. The two women may be the same age and body build, each having the same size cyst on the right ovary, but their responses can vary drastically.

Ruby comes for a routine visit during which I discover that she has a cyst. I ask her, "Have you had pain in your abdomen or pelvis or noticed that something just didn't feel right?"

"No, I haven't noticed anything unusual or had any pain. Everything seems fine."

An hour later I see Pearl, who is complaining of severe pain. "You have to do something," she says. "Nothing I have taken has relieved the pain."

Both Ruby and Pearl have benign (nonmalignant) ovarian cysts, which means that at the time of ovulation, a fluid-filled, blisterlike structure forms on the surface of the ovary. The vast majority of these resolve without treatment other than observation and something given for pain. That is the course I follow with Ruby. But because of the severity of Pearl's complaint, I eventually do laparoscopic surgery to remove the cyst from her ovary.

Another common example is the pain associated with menstruation, called dysmenorrhea. Most women learn about their periods from their mothers. If a woman's mother has taught her that menstruation will be painful or unbearable, and if the mother continually complains about her own menstrual pain, the daughter is much more likely to experience problems with dysmenorrhea. Likewise, a woman whose mother has dealt matter-of-factly with menstrual pain will be more able to cope with such pain.

Different people respond to the same apparent degree of pain in different ways. Some of this has to do with each person's "pain threshold," but some of it has to do with learned responses to painful stimuli. Some people depend on their own will and internal resources to combat pain, while others resort to medication to manage their pain. This doesn't mean that there isn't real pain in the first case; a different reaction to pain is simply evident in each case.

Having pain may be an indicator of illness, but it may also be a reflection of one's emotional state. It is possible to complain of pain and yet have no detectable physical pathology. Nevertheless, pain should always be investigated to rule out organic disease before further assessment is made of a person's physical and emotional health.

What Is Health?

Everyone lives on a continuum between health and illness. Even those presumed to be in the very best state of wellness may have an underlying malady that will eventually result in symptomatic disease. Given the right set of circumstances, exposure to certain bacteria or viruses, subtle changes in the immune defense mechanisms, or contact with environmental toxins or carcinogens, the seemingly impervious shells we live in can become victims of an uncompromising assault. The result can be physical and/or emotional illness that effects significant changes in our lives.

Because of this uncertainty, fear of illness is a universal concern. People in all societies feel an ever present uneasiness about disease and its potential for personal, familial, and social devastation. In addition, women live with concerns unique to their gender:

infertility, pregnancy, and complications related to pregnancy;

menstrual disorders;

benign conditions of the uterus, which may cause pain
   and abnormal bleeding;
cancer of the breast, ovary, uterus, and cervix;
depression and premenstrual syndrome;
stress-related disorders, which are more prevalent in
   women than in men.

With our extraordinary emphasis in the West on medical knowledge and scientific research and because dramatic advances have been made in recent decades, many
people tend to equate *health* with what can be measured
by a physician or a laboratory. This view of health fails to
take into account the importance of emotional and spiritual health. In reality, much more is involved in the meaning of health than what we can see or test. We could diagram a more holistic view of health by drawing a circle and
labeling slices of the pie as the factors that contribute toward
total health. Or we might draw streams of water cascading
over a waterfall into the river of health below (fig. 1).

In figure 2, I placed the spiritual in the center of a wheel,
because I believe it is the hub around which all other fac-

Figure 1
River Model of Health

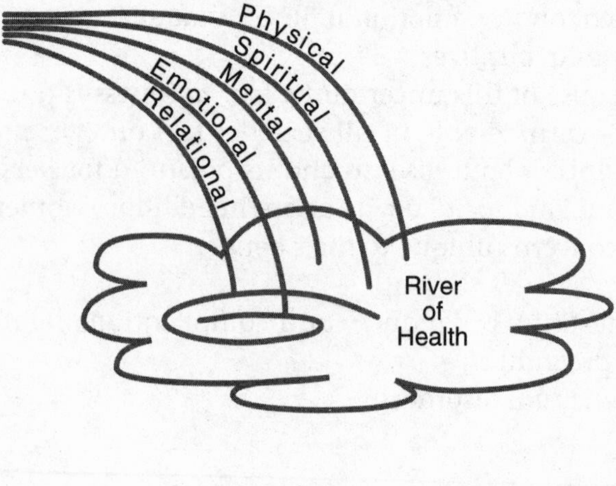

tors rotate. However, each of us has our own way of visualizing health. How you see it is significant, so take a piece of paper and draw your personal visualization of health. The placement, order, and dominance of the factors you select indicate how you approach the matter of your health and that of your family.

Figure 2
Wheel Drawing of Total Health

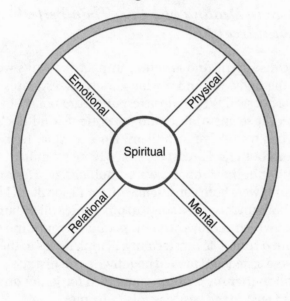

Although we like to talk about holistic health, we tend to divide it into physical, emotional, and spiritual segments for greater ease in thinking about it. Yet, even as we divide it here, you need to remember that all the dimensions influence each other and interact within you in more ways than you probably realize. We have separate ways of dealing with these different areas and distinct professionals we call for help in each, but what we often lack is the coordinating factor or person or even the realization that we need to see all of these as working together to produce the level of total health that we enjoy or desire.

It is often much easier to think of health primarily in physical terms. Medical doctors have so many remedies available—and are often too ready to prescribe a pill instead of taking the time to find out what is really wrong emotionally and spiritually.

Factors in Dealing with Less Than Perfect Physical Health

Because spirit and emotion impact the ways we deal with the body, we find a wide variety of responses when people get sick. When those responses are not easily categorized, it seems frightening for patients and doctors to even begin to delve into them. For example, Jenny and Barbara both had breast cancer. When I examined them, I found that their cancers were small in size. Their mammograms were both consistent with small, localized lesions. They both underwent a surgical procedure called "lumpectomy," which removes the mass and surrounding tissue without a complete mastectomy. Lymph nodes in the armpits were tested and proved negative for metastatic cancer. Radiation therapy was recommended for Jenny and Barbara to ensure the best possible outcome.

Jenny decided that she was not going to succumb to the disease. She faced the diagnosis, entered radiation therapy with determination, and refused to allow the disease to keep her from living her normal life. Barbara, on the other hand, was devastated by the diagnosis, became deeply depressed, and initially refused to accept radiation. Her manner of responding to the diagnosis resulted in emotional problems for her and caused a disruption in her marriage.

The Patient's Attitude

What was the difference between Jenny and Barbara? Many factors, of course, but one of the most key was *attitude*. Some women are not naturally fighters; when faced with difficult circumstances, they do not feel that they can overcome. Usually the disease gets the best of them. Those who fight the obstacles may not always be cured, but often they are not as devastated by their disease.

Jenny and Barbara had different views of health. Jenny acted as if she was healthy, because she didn't see her illness as an obstacle large enough to keep her from living as well as possible. Barbara acted as if she was not going to be healthy, because she allowed the disease to interfere with her other areas of wellness.

I am not suggesting that you shouldn't grieve or be concerned when you are told that you have an illness. But you need to take charge of the situation and process the information given to you by healthcare providers. Then you need to make educated decisions about your health management. After you have done this, you can better control your feelings and expectations for the future. If you expect the worst about a situation, you may get it. If you tend to expect the best and can place the future in God's loving providence, you will be better able to move on with your life, hoping that the medical care you have chosen and your faith in God will bring the best possible outcome.

Because our culture emphasizes the scientific so strongly in our approach to health, we need to pay particular attention to religious attitudes—an aspect of total health that is only recently receiving wide attention. Americans are a highly religious people who frequently participate in religious healing activities, such as praying about their health or watching and attending faith-healing services. In a survey of 203 hospitalized patients, 94 percent believed that spiritual health is as important as physical health; 73 percent reported praying daily; 58 percent had strong religious beliefs; 42 percent had attended faith-healing services.[1]

In spite of such strong religious belief in the general public, medical practitioners frequently neglect the faith of their patients. In the above survey, 80 percent of the patients said their physicians rarely or never addressed spiritual issues, 77 percent believed they should, and 48 percent desired their physicians to pray with them; 42 percent wanted their physicians to ask them about their faith-healing experiences.[2] In a separate study of 146 family physicians and 135 family practice patients, only 11 percent of the physicians said they frequently addressed religious issues with patients, while 40 percent of the patients thought their providers should discuss these issues. The study showed that significantly more patients than physicians believed in God.[3]

Your religious commitment plays a significant role in your physical and emotional well-being. Studies have confirmed this influence in such diverse areas as: happiness, life satisfaction, marital adjustment, self-esteem, moral values, anxiety about death, coping with medical illness, stresses in life, caregiving, degree of control, better health-care utilization, overall wellness, substance abuse, juvenile delinquency, and sexual activity outside of marriage. Your degree of religiousness and your perception of God affect your sense of loneliness; if you see God as helpful, you will feel less lonely, whereas if you see Him as wrathful, you will be more lonely.[4] Many people believe that being married and attending church regularly affect their health.[5] Studies such as these indicate that persons perceive that they are not only healthier when they are religious but that they fare better in healthcare outcomes.

In spite of these data, many people continue to attribute illness to external factors rather than to things that are going on within. Even in a study of psychiatric patients, where you might think respondents would be more likely to recognize internal factors as the cause of illness, 81 percent attributed their illnesses to external factors rather than to their emotional or spiritual state.[6] People cry to God for healing when they become ill, but they fail to look within to see what might be wrong emotionally and spiritually that could be causing disease.

The Doctor's Attitude

We have increasing evidence that the attitude of a doctor toward a patient influences the person's response clinically. If your doctor conveys to you that you are ill and does not offer you encouragement, you are much more likely to lose hope, be sick longer, or not recover at all. Unfortunately, most in the medical profession do not utilize these data to influence their practice of medicine. In medical school we were taught that talking about the spiritual with patients is inappropriate. In addition, many physicians are embarrassed to discuss spiritual issues with their patients, perhaps because they fear the questions they might be asked or that a patient might request that the doctor pray for him or her.

Studies have indicated that health professionals tend to be less religious in a traditional sense than the general public. A 1990 sample of 409 clinical psychologists showed that only 4 percent believed in a personal, transcendent God; 18 percent believed that organized religion was the primary source of their spirituality; and 51 percent described their spiritual path as "alternative" and "not part of organized religion."[7] In a 1991 study of family physicians, researchers found that 64 percent believed in God, 45 percent believed in the afterlife, 60 percent prayed, and 43 percent felt close to God.[8]

The attitude of your physician influences the relationship the two of you have, and that relationship affects the confidence you have in your doctor as a person who is able to effect a cure. If you believe your doctor doesn't think you are healthy, you will probably rate yourself as being unhealthy, but the opposite is also true.

Geneva was a middle-aged mother of three, who came to see me one month after I delivered her grandson. She had not had a pelvic exam in seven years. Because her mother had died of ovarian cancer when Geneva was twenty-eight, she did not like to go to doctors, fearing that she might have the same problem.

I took Geneva's history and performed a physical examination, which indicated she had an enlarged right ovary. An ultrasound scan of the pelvis revealed a suspicious, seven-centimeter ovarian mass, which required surgery. During surgery, Geneva was found to have a Stage II ovarian cancer, with a predicted survival rate for five years of 50 percent. We were able to remove all of the cancer, but the fluid in the abdominal cavity tested positive for malignant cells. Chemotherapy was recommended in an attempt to eradicate any remaining malignant cells.

Geneva was very depressed when she was informed of her diagnosis after the surgery. She reminded me of her mother's death and said, "I know that I'm going to die. I don't want to be miserable with the side effects of chemotherapy like hair loss and nausea, so please don't ask me to take it."

"Geneva," I responded, "I understand your grief and your reluctance to be treated with anticancer drugs, but remember, there is more involved here than just how you may feel while you are being treated. You have a husband, three daughters, two sons-in-law, and a new grandchild to think of. They need you and want you to do everything you can to survive. You are also important to your friends, your church, and your community." Geneva went ahead with the treatment.

Betty was quite a different story. I heard about her case from her sister, who is my patient. Betty had been diagnosed with ovarian cancer of a slightly better stage than Geneva's. Her doctor had told her about chemotherapy, its risks and benefits. When Betty expressed reservations about treatment, he told her just to wait and see what would happen. Betty had evidence of recurrence within one year and was dead fifteen months after her first diagnosis.

Encouragement from competent physicians, as well as their faith and prayers, can make all the difference in the world!

The Patient's Personality Type

Sometimes, in spite of reassurance from a doctor, a patient may convince herself that she is ill and nothing will dissuade her from that.

When Susan came to me for a gynecological evaluation, she quickly told me that she was afraid she was going to die from cancer. Her maternal grandmother, who was a heavy smoker, had died of lung cancer, and her mother had died of cervical cancer when she was only forty-five. Susan had two sisters who were both healthy, but she believed she was the one who would get cancer.

I did a thorough examination and found everything to be normal. The lab studies showed nothing to cause alarm. At Susan's insistence, I ordered an ultrasound scan of the pelvis and a chest X ray, and both of these were also normal. Susan had smoked for several years, and during this time of anxiety, her habit had increased to two packs a day. I strongly advised her to stop, but she said she couldn't right now. I prescribed a quit-smoking class and nicotine patches to help her, but she took advantage of neither. Her anxiety continued to increase until she required psychiatric care on an outpatient basis.

After that visit, I didn't see Susan for a long time. About three years later, as I was reviewing the operating room schedule before my day in surgery, I noticed her name on the list. She was scheduled for a bronchoscopy by one of the chest surgeons. This procedure uses a lighted instrument to look into the large airways to the lungs and do a biopsy if needed. I later found out that the biopsy was positive for cancer of the lung. Susan had a portion of her lung removed and underwent chemotherapy, but the cancer was advanced at the time of diagnosis, and she died two years later.

Of course, cigarette smoking was the most likely cause of the lung cancer. But I believe Susan's obsession with cancer and her conviction that she had it played a role in her demise. If she had not been so stressed because of her belief that she would die of cancer, she might have been able to stop smoking.

Physicians have now identified the type C personality as being more frequently associated with cancer. People of this type possess pathological niceness, an inability to express their true feelings, and a great deal of repressed anger. Patients with a phobia about illness need to be shown by their physicians that they are truly free of disease. They also need help identifying those aspects of their personality that may predispose them to malignancies or other stress-related diseases.[9]

In Search of Good Health

We know the best therapy for any disease is prevention. A balanced diet, appropriate exercise, good hygiene, avoidance of harmful substances, and regular medical evaluations are essential to the maintenance of good health. Yet even with the best preventive techniques, acute or chronic illness may strike and leave a patient wondering, "Why did this happen to me?"

People of all faiths tend to associate physical disease with spiritual malady. This seems especially perplexing for Christians, because we are taught that God wants the very best for us. If He does, how can He allow such bad things to happen to good people?

In the Gospel of John we read of a man who had something bad happen to him, leaving him crippled for thirty-eight years (John 5:1–15). One Sabbath, Jesus healed this man. Later they met in the temple, and Jesus reminded the man that he was healed. Then He said, "See, you are well again. Stop sinning or something worse may happen to you" (John 5:14). Many use this verse to suggest that sin causes disease, but that is not what Jesus said. Rather, He was reminding the man that sinful or self-destructive behavior has consequences; these might include illness or death.

Disease is a fact of life in a fallen world, and yet we have a choice as to how we will view it. Instead of seeing it as a punishment because we aren't sufficiently spiritual, as a test from God to determine whether we will persevere, as a curse from God upon us and our families, or as a punishment for our sin, we can choose to regard illness as an opportunity for God to reveal His power in and through us. When we are ill, we should ask, "God, what do You want to teach me through this experience?" We can pray that healing will come in God's good time and manner.

Living with Stress

Our health can be profoundly influenced by the amount of stress with which we live. Stress comes from three sources: our environment, our body, and our thoughts. Figure 3

illustrates the effects of stress on our lives. When the wires
hang loosely, peace, calm, and relaxation maintain a
healthy stability. But when the wires are strung too tightly,
stress, anxiety, and tension bend the poles toward an unstable state of illness.

Figure 3

Tension Model of health and Illness

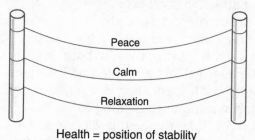

Health = position of stability

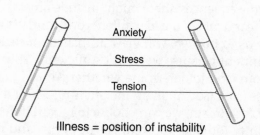

Illness = position of instability

If *health* were nothing more than your physical condition, then *healing* would mean finding a remedy for whatever ails your body. However, the majority of illnesses entering hospitals and doctors' offices in the United States are
related to factors other than physical. Those other factors
may have contributed to the physical condition the patients
now complain of, but they are not physical in themselves.

Dr. Juliet Schor indicates that 30 percent of all adults
admit to high levels of stress. One in every ten Americans

suffers from an anxiety-related disorder. Three-fourths of all American women have at least one tension headache each month.[10] Appropriate levels of stress can serve as valuable motivators to achieve great things or make important decisions. But when the stress results in physical illness, you need to change your situation in order to protect your health. Some doctors believe that as much as 70 percent of illness is ultimately stress-related.[11]

In our book, *Stress and the Woman's Body*, Linda and I discuss the effects of stress on the woman's body.[12] Disorders such as fibromyalgia, irritable bowel syndrome, tension headaches, eating disorders, premenstrual syndrome, menstrual disorders, and more are described. When a woman's negative stressors exceed her positive adaptors to stress, disease can result. When the stress is not dealt with or dissipated, it is often internalized, resulting in the release of hormonal substances that cause abnormal function or disease. This is one reason spiritual and emotional well-being are so critical to physical health.

What Is Healing?

To decide what you mean by *healing*, you need to know what you mean by *health*. As you recall the diagram you drew of health, you might want to attach some rough percentages to the various elements of health or illness. For instance, do you consider physical health or illness to be 20 percent of total health, or 50 or 80 percent? How does emotional health compare with spiritual? Over what factors do you have a large measure of control?

All too often people seek healing, even pray for healing, with only a vague idea of what they are asking. Or they may seek healing for something they could cure or prevent themselves.

As you consider what you think healing is, ask yourself what would make you feel that you are in total health or completely healed. Would it include your emotions, your relationships, your work, your hopes? What would you need to change, to eliminate, to begin, to forgive? For you, does healing involve a miracle, medical intervention, or both? (We will think more about this in chapter 11.) As you consider your total health, let me make a few suggestions—things I'm sure you have heard before but which you may see in a different way in the context of this chapter.

- Be sure you are on a spiritual journey with God. Learn to repent of your sins to God and then confess to those you have wronged. Remember that unconfessed sin can cause anxiety and guilt, and these can lead to spiritual and physical disease. Study God's Word and seek what He has for you in both personal and group Bible study. Spend much time in prayer and also consider the discipline of fasting. Develop your own quiet time with the Lord, and honor that time as a priority. Pour out your heart to God, telling Him your anxieties and concerns, but also spend time praising Him for all He has done for you and others. Also learn how to listen to God and to His people. Begin sharing your joy and concerns with others. Encouraging others and asking about their joys and problems will get your mind off of your own problems.
- Regarding your physical health, find a truly healthy diet—one that is low in fat and sugar but with adequate fibers, grains, and fluids. You can obtain a dietary guide from any clinic or at your library; the hard part is sticking with it. Try to maintain your weight rather than going up and down. Stay away from fad diets and weight-loss pills. The key to weight reduction is to modify your behavior so that you rec-

ognize food as a source of energy rather than something to make you feel good about yourself.

- You may not like to exercise, but you can't afford not to. You need regular aerobic exercise for at least thirty minutes three to four times a week in order to control your weight and maintain your energy level.
- Stay away from harmful substances, including nicotine, drugs, alcohol, caffeine, and any foods to which you feel addicted.
- For a sense of emotional health, you need to love and feel loved. Spend time developing relationships that are important to you with both family and friends. Emotional health involves facing your dark side and dealing with difficult issues, rather than shelving them for some future time. Find ways to deal with the stresses in your life and learn to say *no* to many of the things in which other people want you to engage. Also, take time for activities that relax and renew you.[13]

God's Design for Healing

After examining the examples of healing described in the Bible, it appears to me that God has designed a definite plan for restoration to wholeness. Healing doesn't always occur in the expected or desired manner, but you must follow the plan if you desire an opportunity for spiritual, physical, emotional, and relational wellness.

Acknowledge your illness. In 2 Kings 5 we are told about the captain of the army of Aram, a foreigner named Naaman who was sent to the king of Israel and then to the prophet Elisha by the king of Aram. Naaman had leprosy and he needed to admit his diseased state to Elisha and humble himself before God before any healing would occur. The first step to wholeness is the admission that you are sick.

Seek God. Although we know that God seeks us and draws us to Himself in the process of salvation, it appears that God expects us to seek Him out in the matter of healing. The woman with the issue of blood might not have been healed had she not sought out the Master and bravely touched the hem of His garment. Sometimes others have to bring the ill to the Lord, as did the friends of the lame man who was lowered through the roof into Jesus' presence. Whatever the type of illness, we must approach God and seek His healing touch.

Do as God directs. In the fifth chapter of John we are told of a man who had been sick for thirty-eight years. He couldn't make it into the pool at Bethesda to seek healing from the waters there because of his lameness. Jesus told the man to take up his pallet and walk, and the man did so in obedience. Naaman, the captain with leprosy, was instructed by Elisha to bathe in the Jordan River seven times. Healing came only when Naaman consented and obeyed. God may direct us to do things that seem unnecessary or inconvenient and He may instruct us to do what we believe is impossible. We must obey to find healing.

Believe by faith that God can heal. The Syrophoenician woman not only pursued Jesus on behalf of her demon-possessed daughter but also believed that He could heal her even from a distance. Faith in God's healing power may exist in someone other than the target of the healing, but someone must have faith.

Trust that healing has occurred or is in process. When Jairus sought the Great Physician on behalf of his dying daughter, he obviously had faith. Even when people came to inform him that his daughter had died, Jairus believed that she was being healed. He trusted Jesus' word that healing was in process, and when he arrived at home, he found his daughter healed as he expected.

Repent of the sin in your life. Jesus told the woman caught in adultery that she was forgiven and that she should leave and sin no more. When Jesus saw the man who had been by the pool at Bethesda, he instructed, "Behold, you have become well; do not sin anymore, so that nothing worse may befall you." Jesus recognized that sin and its effects create guilt and sickness of the heart that may result in persistent illness and interfere with the opportunity for wholeness.

Trust in God's timing. Lazarus's resurrection from the dead reminds us that God's timing is always perfect when it comes to healing. We may not like it or have the patience to wait for God's time, but He not only knows how to heal, but when to heal. He knows how rapidly the process should progress and precisely when we are ready for healing.

Give Him praise. In Luke 17 Jesus healed ten lepers of their disease. In obedience to Jesus and in accordance with Jewish law, they went to the high priest to have their healing confirmed. When all was said and done, only one returned to praise Jesus for the healing. Jesus asked, "Was no one found who turned back to give glory to God, except this foreigner?" This former leper was informed that his faith had made him whole. God expects our praise and thanksgiving when healing occurs.

These are not magical steps or rituals necessary for the procurement of physical healing. They are precepts from God's Word that describe for us what we must do to find wholeness in Him. Each must occur before true, complete healing may take place.

Jesus and Your Health

As you have read the stories of Jesus' interaction with women who needed healing, you have seen how He defined health as more than physical. His attention to what we call *spiritual* also included their lifestyles. As He moved to heal or restore to life, He demonstrated deep compassion for family members who were grieving or dealing with potential loss. Jesus was never harsh with women; He seemed to desire that they be comforted as well as healed. Yet this was not a mindless comfort, but one in which they began to see His purposes for them now and into the future.

When Jesus began His public ministry, He shocked the populace with His complete lack of concern for customs that forbade men to publicly interact with women. Neither gender nor social status hindered the love of God that came embodied in Jesus. He saw people at heart level, and His empathy for women and their social condition placed a radical new significance on their lives. The fact that He healed women indicated that He recognized them as equal in importance to men. He encouraged, transformed, and forgave these women, just as He had the men. He even appeared first to a woman after He was raised from the dead (see Matt. 28:8–10; John 20:10–18).

Jesus was always prepared to heal, because He was constantly in touch with His Father. In time alone with God, He prepared Himself in prayer and fasting. We need to learn from Him and prepare ourselves in these same ways. Healing comes from truly being delivered from the self that wants to focus on what we can get from God and being converted into persons more interested in being what God is calling us to be and doing what He is calling us to do for others.

John Newton was one person so converted and changed. Before he came to Christ, he was a slave dealer. After his conversion, he became a clergyman and a poet. In his majestic hymn, "Glorious Things of Thee Are Spoken," there is a little-known verse that contains a wonderful line about God raising people from self with His love so that they can reign with Him. This is not just a someday hope; it can be your experience now.

> Blest inhabitants of Zion, washed in the Redeemer's blood!
> Jesus, whom their souls rely on, makes them kings and
> priests to God.
> 'Tis his love his people raises over self to reign as kings,
> And as priests, his solemn praises each for a thank offering
> brings.

Jesus still reaches out with unconditional love and concern for your total self. He still blends physical healing with restoration of emotional and spiritual wholeness. He wants to relate to you this way. He knows your pain, your tears, and your sorrows, and He is reaching out to you, just as He did so long ago, with love, healing, and promise. He came to earth as the Savior, which means Redeemer/Healer. You can choose to let Him be the restorer of your life, the healer of your innermost self, the health of your body and emotions.

eleven

The Power of Prayer

*M*ajor changes are taking place in health care today. Part of this is due to rising costs and restrictions from insurance companies. But many of the changes are the result of a search for a more holistic approach to healing. This search has led millions of people to seek help in alternative therapies.

To better see these changes in perspective, we need to remember that what we call *traditional medicine* is relatively new. The American Medical Association was formed as recently as 1846 in response to the 1844 formation of the American Institute of Homeopathy.

Homeopathic medicine uses natural substances in the belief that the body can heal itself. In the nineteenth century it remained strong, but it fell out of favor early in this century. By 1940 all of the twenty-two schools of medicine had closed, and by 1970 only 150 practitioners remained. However, in the past few decades there has been a resurgence of interest in these therapies as well as in many other alternative therapies. Today about three thousand

155

homeopathic practitioners work in the United States; many of them are medically trained. There is also strong support in Europe for this approach to treatment.[1]

As we have looked back to Jesus' approach to illness, we must of course remember that physicians of His time had no knowledge of what we take for granted as standard medical practice. In fact, almost everything they did might be labeled *alternative* by today's physicians.

One of the alternative practices in which medical people have increasing interest today is prayer in its various forms. A good deal of research has been done to test the effect of prayer and other religious practices on health in general and specifically on recovery from disease and surgery. This research is in part a response to the religious beliefs of the general public and their disaffection with the way most medical people ignore their beliefs. In 1996, *Time* magazine funded a telephone survey of 1,004 persons to inquire about the relation of health and prayer. Some of the questions and responses were:[2]

	Yes	No
Do you believe in the healing power of personal prayer?	82%	13%
Do you believe praying for someone else can help cure their illness?	73%	21%
Do you believe doctors should join their patients in prayer, if the patients request it?	64%	27%

Increasing numbers of medical people are advocating the validity of prayer as part of a holistic approach to health. Dr. Herbert Benson, president of the Mind/Body Medical Institute of Boston's Deaconess Hospital and Harvard Medical School, is one of the leaders in this field. He estimates that between 60 and 90 percent of visits to doctors are in "the mind-body, stress-related realm," chronic diseases against which "traditional modes of therapy—pharmaceutical and surgical—don't work well."[3]

In his recent book, *Timeless Healing,* Dr. Benson writes about the "faith factor," the combined force of two internal influences—"remembered wellness and the elicitation of the relaxation response. But it became clear that a person's religious convictions or life philosophy enhanced the average effects of the relaxation response." As Dr. Benson explored the combination of spirituality and health, he discovered that "women had higher spirituality scores than men, for reasons we don't yet understand."[4]

Dr. Benson believes that faith in God is good for people, as are many kinds of group religious experiences and rituals, including prayer. He advocates trusting one's instincts more and applying "self-care." By this he means to work with medical people as well as with your own lifestyle to achieve maximum health. "This includes mind/body reactions such as remembered wellness, the relaxation response and the faith factor. It also embraces good nutrition, exercise and other means of stress management."[5]

Why Research Prayer?

Some people may wonder why doctors and hospitals are beginning to carefully research whether prayer works. It is important to remember that these projects are for the purpose of validating a nonscientific activity—prayer—for the scientific world. While many doctors may know the value of prayer in a personal sense, they want to see it demonstrated and validated in controlled studies. *Time* magazine reports several findings:

> According to a 1995 Dartmouth study, one of the strongest predictors of survival after open-heart

surgery is the degree to which patients say they draw
strength and comfort from religion.

Thirty years of research on blood pressure show that
churchgoers have lower blood pressure than nonchurchgoers.

Those who attend church regularly have half the risk
of dying from coronary-artery disease as those who
rarely go to church.

Churchgoers suffer from fewer anxiety-related illnesses
and have lower rates of depression.

People who are involved in both church and social
groups have a fourteen-fold advantage in main-
taining good health over those who are isolated or
lack faith.[6]

In a report on prayer research, Michael E. McCullough
states that "the primary goal of Christian prayer is not to
improve one's health—it is to commune with God. . . . Prayer
is an act of 'self-dedication rather than self-seeking.'" He
suggests three pathways for the prayer/health link:

Prayer may change the ways that individuals appraise
stressful events.

Prayer may activate health-promotive psychological
mechanisms such as structure, meaning, and hope.

Prayer . . . may involve neuroimmunological, cardiovascular, and brain electrical changes, and muscle
relaxation.[7]

As I have examined the data, I find that more than 250
studies indicate that religious persons are generally
healthier than nonreligious people. Also, about 130 studies conclude that prayer is effective in promoting healing.
This healing may occur in all kinds of persons, but it happens more frequently in those who have faith and who
attend church.

The Mystery of Healing

While I am delighted about the renewed interest in prayer in relation to healing, I know that healing is and always will be a profound mystery. I am sure that God heals, but I am also sure that He will not be manipulated by us.

When we pray for healing for ourselves or others, we need to pray for the whole person, not just for one physical symptom. God wants to make us whole in His time and in His way. When people are not healed by our definition of that word, we must not assume that they did not receive grace from God or that He does not love them. We all know people who have experienced redemptive power in the midst of their suffering.

No matter how many times an individual is healed, the day will come when there is no more physical healing, and the body will die. That last physical failure, death, is hidden behind a veil. In our lack of understanding about death, we are sometimes tempted to speculate and even to follow some of the current teachings from those who claim that they have gone to the other side and returned. While we do not know how reliable these after-death experiences are, we do know that we can trust the issues of life and death into God's hands. It is not necessary that we be able to define what He has chosen to retain to Himself.

Julie and Brian's story illustrates the mystery that surrounds the issues of life and death and also our lack of control over so much that affects us. Julie and Brian were in their early thirties when they came to see me because of fertility problems. In their previous city, they had undergone extensive testing to determine the cause of their inability to conceive. By the time they came to me, they were to the point of pursuing in-vitro fertilization techniques.

For many years they had prayed for a child and had been supported in prayer by their family and members of their church. After we had attempted in-vitro fertilization three times, Julie and Brian were exhausted from the strain and also somewhat angry, and they decided that a change of scenery would do them good.

During their vacation in the Caribbean, they conceived. Some weeks after their return, Julie came to see me for a blood pregnancy test that was indeed positive. The couple was thrilled and began to call their families and friends and to make preparations for their long-awaited baby. During the next months, Julie was evaluated with routine laboratory work and an ultrasound scan. All of her testing was normal, and the pregnancy progressed smoothly.

When the baby was full term, Julie went into labor spontaneously. Although the baby had some fetal heart-rate problems during labor, Julie was able to deliver vaginally. With great anticipation, Brian watched as Julie pushed her daughter from the birth canal and into my waiting hands. As soon as I positioned her in my arms to cut the umbilical cord, I was aware that something was wrong. The baby's extremities were shortened, and her neck and chest were unusually broad. She had some difficulty breathing, and I had to place a tube into her larynx so that I could ventilate her. A neonatologist was called, and the baby was whisked off to the neonatal intensive care unit for stabilization.

For several days little Karen teetered on the brink of life and death. Julie and Brian and their families were distraught. It became obvious that Karen had a form of dwarfism and perhaps other developmental anomalies.

I spent a good deal of time with the couple over the next few days talking, praying, and crying together. After five days Karen began to improve, and the reality of having a child with major congenital defects began to set in. Both parents were very upset, but Brian was especially angry.

"We trusted God for a miracle, and look what He did for us! Now He's going to have to work a miracle in us."

I tried to be compassionate and understanding, but it became increasingly evident that Brian was rejecting the child as his own and beginning to blame Julie for the baby's defects. After several days, I sat down with them in a quiet room and said, "Brian and Julie, I don't know why God gave you Karen in the way that He did after all your years of trying to have a baby. But I do know that you must be very special people, or He wouldn't have put her in your care. You see, although Karen may appear on the exterior to be handicapped, God doesn't look at the outside. He looks at the heart, and I'm certain that Karen is a very special person on the inside."

The next day Julie called me and said, "Dr. Hager, you were so right. Brian and I have been feeling sorry for ourselves instead of being concerned about Karen. As we talked about her defects, we were reminded of our frailty before God. We knelt together and asked God to forgive us and to thank Him for giving us Karen. We know it won't be easy, but we are confident that He will give us the strength to see this through. Thank you for your prayers."

Even in the midst of grief and anguish, God is ever present. He understands our despair and also our anger. He never gives a burden greater than we can bear, and He promises to be with us in every trial.

Karen is now three years old. I talked with Julie recently, and she said that raising their child has been a real challenge but that they are both learning valuable lessons about loving unconditionally and are depending on God to supply all of their needs. She also told me that Karen's loving personality has brought them closer to the heart of God.

Toward a Theology of Healing

That God heals—of this I am fully certain. However, when, why, how, and under what specific circumstances, by what virtue, or in satisfaction of what requirement—about these I have no certain answers, nor do I believe anyone else does. Also, it is impossible for us to determine whether God is most desirous of working toward our physical health or our emotional and spiritual health at any given time.

We cannot understand God by looking only at His healing acts. However, we can bring some degree of order to our theology of healing by looking to God and fixing our minds on what the Word reveals to us of His unchanging character and nature. We make a grave error when we try to interpret God through our circumstances. Rather, we must interpret our circumstances by looking at God.

Any examination of healing needs to begin with a willingness to embrace the mystery and to own our utter incapability of manipulating God and His healing power according to our desires. Any theology of healing must include the redemptive power that can be inherent in suffering and the inescapable truth that we do not understand death and dying. The veil is impenetrable from this side, and apparently that is the way God wants it to be. Death is either the very worst or the very best thing ever to happen to the human race. Maybe it is both.

Most of us would prefer a definition of healing in which we or our loved ones are restored to complete health on this side of eternity. However, the scriptural approach is to put our total well-being into the hands of the One who made us. That means surrendering our choices as well as those influences over which we have no control. It may also mean acknowledging and confessing some things about ourselves that we have tried to hide, because the physical, emotional, and spiritual cannot be separated.

I believe God enables healthcare professionals to be a part of the healing process, but I know that we are only instruments available for His use. Because of this, I never feel I am less of a professional when I ask patients and their families to pray for healing or when I offer to pray for them. Many doctors resist the notion of praying for healing, but once they do recognize the great power of God and realize it is available to them as they try to help their patients, they can enter into a partnership that includes patient, medical knowledge, a doctor's compassion, and the power of God.

A crucially important factor to remember about prayer and healing relates to timing. We always want healing to occur on our timetable—immediately. Yet we saw in the stories of Jesus' healing miracles that sometimes He delayed. We don't understand His delays any more than did the people of His time, but we know that He does not forget us. Instead, He has another plan—one beyond our vision—for achieving wholeness.

Dr. Larry Dossey's book, *Healing Words: The Power of Prayer and the Practice of Medicine,* considers the relationship of prayer and healing. He asks, "Why examine prayer in healing? It works!" As he looks to the future, Dr. Dossey writes, "Prayer will become incorporated into the mainstream for healing. So pervasive will its use become that NOT to recommend the use of prayer as an integral part of medical care will one day constitute medical malpractice."[8]

Churches and Healing Prayers

In churches of many different persuasions, prayers for healing are again taking their place where they belong, as part of the local ministry to believers and in the context of pastoral care, preaching and teaching, the sacraments, and the fellowship of Christians who know and love each other. There is better chance for healing in the local church community than in an impersonal setting where practitioners know nothing of the individual.

Prayers for healing in local churches take different forms. One of the most common is the prayer chain, in which people on a phone list are quickly alerted when there is a need in the congregation. Another form is the scheduled healing prayer service, perhaps during the week or following a Sunday service. Or the prayers for healing may happen during the primary service of the week, as people feel free to come to the front, perhaps during communion or after the benediction, to receive individual prayer. Another form this may take is when elders and clergy go to a home or hospital to pray for and anoint one who is sick. However, the practice of anointing and praying should not be only in the home or hospital. It belongs back in the church as part of a total ministry.

This renewed practice stems from Jesus' healing ministry and also from these verses in James:

> Is any one of you in trouble? He should pray. Is anyone happy? Let him sing songs of praise. Is any one of you sick? He should call the elders of the church to pray over him and anoint him with oil in the name of the Lord. And the prayer offered in faith will make the sick person well; the Lord will raise him up. If he has sinned, he will be forgiven. Therefore confess your sins to each other and pray for each other so that you may be healed. The prayer of a righteous man is powerful and effective.
>
> James 5:13–16

When a church desires to inaugurate this type of public ministry, there should be some explanation to the congregation so that they will understand what is happening. They need to be assured that their requests will be held in confidence. They also need to understand that they should not command God to perform instant miracles. This is where the idea of total health is so important; those who are prayed for may gradually move toward wholeness rather than experience instantaneous healing.

A church member recently said that he would have faith if he saw a miracle. The elder offering the healing prayers responded, "There is something even greater than a miracle—we can teach our children and young people that they can come to God in every circumstance, for every need, and know He listens and cares for them. If they can come to believe this for the rest of their lives, that is so much more than one instantaneous miracle. If you can exercise your faith, you will see miracles, perhaps not in the manner of time you envision, but He will heal in His time."

There is another important aspect about praying for one another in the local church—it pictures the corporate life of the body of Christ. The apostle Paul wrote so much about the way we are joined together to be Christ's body in the world, and yet we often see little evidence of this in church circles. To pray together for physical, emotional, or spiritual healing is to place ourselves in a totally dependent position before the One who is the Head of the body.

Of course, it is fully appropriate for you to ask your medical professionals to pray with you when you are ill. If they seem uncomfortable with this, don't press the issue, but you might find more openness than you expect. Some medical schools are now incorporating spiritual training into their curriculum. One school near Chicago recently announced that medical students would be working with chaplains for a year to learn how to pray with their patients.

Pastors need to learn to work with doctors in praying for healing. The doctors can help pastors understand the specific physical problems so that their prayers can be more focused. The pastors, in turn, can help doctors learn how to pray. As they work together, they may benefit just as much as their patients and parishioners.

Another aspect of healing prayer with significant possibilities is to enlist people who are sick to pray for others with similar maladies. We usually think of the well praying for the sick, and yet who can better understand the needs of those in distress than others who are also suffering? Sometimes this kind of prayer leads to the formation of support groups for those with particular illnesses. When those who are sick pray for others, they tend to break through their own fear of illness as well as the isolation that can cut them off from others. Sometimes those praying also experience a dramatic betterment in their own health, which again underlines the unity of body, mind, emotion, and spirit.

twelve

Behind the Office Door

*j*ust as you are unique, so is every woman who comes in my office door. The story each one tells as I take her history reveals much more than the medical facts that have brought her to see me. If I could sit down with you and hear your story, it too would reveal a lot more than a simple medical record.

Any seasoned physician knows that relieving a patient's symptoms and treating the underlying problem may involve two entirely different approaches. As a scientist, I am interested in the presenting medical problem. I have been trained to observe the body systems and look for the source of the complaint. Perhaps I recommend a surgical procedure, or a simple course of a powerful antibiotic may be all that is needed. But even the most potent drug and most skilled surgical technique cannot always bring healing to a patient, especially when 60 to 90 percent of visits are stress-related. Often the emotions that run like a hidden stream beneath the surface of the disease play a far more significant role in total healing than anything a doctor can do for the patient. Let's walk through a typical day at the office, and you will see what I mean.

Monday Morning at the Clinic

When I arrive at the office, my assistant tells me that our first patient is Leigh, who is coming for her yearly exam. I delivered two of Leigh and Henry's three children, and over the years her exams have been routine.

As I enter the room, I extend my hand to Leigh and greet her warmly with a smile and the usual questions about her family. I see fatigue in her eyes, and her answers to my questions reveal the source of her weariness. She tells me that she is now working full-time to help with college expenses for their oldest child. The two younger ones still at home have many extra activities, and Leigh has to juggle the demands of her job with those of her family. She feels as if she is running a race she can never win, and guilt is her constant companion. She says, "I love my family, but I feel as if they are sucking the life out of me. No one seems to understand." Although she doesn't say so, I know Leigh wonders if I can do anything to help.

My next patient, Jane, is here for a routine physical and a Pap smear, but before we begin, she wants to ask me a few questions. She has been coming to my office for several years, and I have always thought of her as a highly responsible and fulfilled person. In her personal life she has never chosen to marry and now devotes much of her free time to her aging mother who lives nearby. Jane's successful career has always seemed to be a source of satisfaction to her, but her comments today reveal a woman who is frightened by the prospects for the future.

"There is such increasing pressure in my company for the bottom line that I don't know how much longer I can handle this. I have been giving 100 percent for several years, and now they want more. Since our firm was acquired by a New York company, we have new managers, and I now work for someone younger and less experienced than I am. I really wonder what is going to happen next. I felt a deep satisfaction in my work for many years and used to get some respect for what I did. But not any more."

Lisa, a single mother, is my next patient. She and her one-year-old baby live with her boyfriend, who is the father of the child. Neither Lisa nor Brad have any real career aspirations or marketable skills with which to support their family. Lisa's parents have taken them in, but I know this situation is less than ideal. Today Lisa has a positive pregnancy test. She is not happy about this news and knows that no one else will be either.

Joan is my 10:30 patient. She and her husband have four children aged three to ten, and since I delivered all of them, I am interested in keeping track of how they are. With obvious pride, she shows me a recent picture of the family, but when I look up at her, I see tears streaming down her face. "It may sound crazy, Dr. Hager, but I'm so lonely!" Her face dissolves in tears as she begins to cry in earnest. "I'm surrounded by people, but I don't have any adults to really talk with. When Greg comes home from work, all he wants to do is collapse into a chair and read the paper or watch TV. He helps put the kids to bed, and he's good about keeping things fixed around the house, but he never wants to talk about anything that interests me. I see a couple of neighbors now and then, but they are busy with their kids just like I am. We go to church, but just getting there is such an effort that it barely seems worth going. I feel as if I'm drying up on the inside. And now, with some added bills we've accumulated, Greg wants me to work part-time. In the right kind of job, I would at least have some adults to talk to, but I want that kind of companionship from Greg. I don't know what to do."

At 11:00 Helen is waiting for me. I have known her for many years and have treated her for stress-related disorders. More recently we have been trying a course of Zoloft to relieve depression. She says, "I have been trying to relax, like you said, and have been taking the medicine, but I still am so stressed out. Also, I've had more abdominal pain recently. There aren't many days in a month when I feel really well, and I know I am letting all this spill over on the family, and they don't like it. What am I going to do?"

Kate is my next appointment. Her chart tells me that she has been here recently, and I wonder what could bring her back so soon. Her complaints are vague, but I sense genuine concern in her voice, even fear. I have learned to respect the intuitive knowledge that most women have about their bodies. Kate says she has a foreboding sense of gloom that she can relate only to her physical health. "Something is wrong, but I don't know what. I hope you can discover what it is." I tell her that I will order blood work and also do an ultrasound scan. These tests will give us something to go on. If we find a problem, Kate's intuitive hunches will have brought her in early enough to begin effective treatment.

A Physician in Process

A typical day in a gynecological office involves much more than physical examinations and Pap smears. My conversations with these patients illustrate something very important. As a physician, I must listen with my heart as well as with my mind. Sometimes this simple kindness will do much more than drugs to strengthen and comfort patients. What they say to me is just as significant as any presenting physical symptoms.

I didn't begin my practice eighteen years ago with this understanding, and it has taken time for me to discover its importance. In medical school, we were taught that the doctor knows best. We were trained to take a history of the present illness and significant past disease problems. We questioned patients in a straightforward manner to obtain answers we could quickly write in their medical charts. We learned how to listen with our ears, but we weren't trained to hear the messages underlying our patients' words.

Consequently, many of us missed the covert signs of emotional distress that could have enabled us to assist patients in reaching a deeper level of well-being. We did not ask questions that might have unmasked the true source of disease, because we were more comfortable with questions that elicited brief answers.

I was a true product of the medical training of my time, but I also had another issue that interfered with my ability to listen effectively—my ego. Being considered an astute diagnostician was vital to my self-esteem as a physician. I felt threatened if a patient already had a good idea of what her problem might be. In addition, I wanted to be in complete control of the therapy. Any patient who did not listen to and explicitly follow my advice I labeled as stubborn and ignorant. After all, why would she choose to come to me for medical care and then fail to trust my suggested course of treatment? I was *the doctor;* I knew what was wrong, and I knew precisely what it would take for her to get better. Case closed.

I know now how wrong I was. And as those harmful attitudes spilled over into my marriage, the Lord began to deal with me about my compulsive need to be in control. The Holy Spirit showed me that the other side of my compulsive need to control was fear. In both my professional and personal life, I was operating out of denial and intimidation. Owning up to those behaviors made me feel shameful and weak. Not owning up to them was putting increasingly large barriers between my wife and me. The marriage we were committed to was not proving very satisfying to either one of us. As long as I lived in denial and fear, I could not own any of my part in the problems we were experiencing. Hidden behind a mask was the real David Hager, who believed that honest self-disclosure would inevitably result in abandonment. Of course the reverse was actually true, but it would take a large deposit of trust on my part to begin my journey out from behind the walls I had so carefully constructed.

I am still a Christian physician in process, but time and God and my patients have been great teachers. I have learned to look first into the eyes of my patients and to silently pray for discernment and wisdom in interpreting what I see and hear. I have learned that the key to diagnosis comes not only in answers to questions about particular symptoms but also in extra comments that are thrown in, phrases that drop off into nothingness, or evasiveness. All of these point me in the direction of the real problem.

How can I help patients like Leigh, Jane, Lisa, Joan, Helen, and Kate? Help begins when I walk in the exam room and turn my attention fully to their individual needs. Several other women may be in the waiting room, and each deserves my full attention, but right now I will focus on just one. I know that each patient's healing ultimately rests in the hands of God. I am thankful for the privilege of assisting Him to some extent with my skills as an obstetrician and gynecologist, but I know that the final outcome will always be a result of His power and mercy.

Questions from the Doctor

As I have talked with women over these many years, I have learned from them that I may need to ask certain types of questions to open up a level of communication that will reveal the real issues in their lives. The following are some of the questions I ask most often. You may have heard them in your interaction with physicians.

Are you content in your present situation?
Are you fulfilled in your work?
If you are unfulfilled, what would it take to enable you to move toward the kind of life you really want?
What do you need most in your life?
Why are you really here today?
Do you have quality communication with your husband and/or friends?
Do you experience satisfying intimacy in your marriage?
Are you safe from harm at home? Are your children safe?
Have you experienced harassment at work?
Do you feel trapped? Are things caving in on you?
Do you cry more often than you laugh?
Before your period, do you feel that something comes and takes control of your mind and body?
Do you have enough time alone to think, study, and pray?
Have you developed techniques to dissipate stress in your life?
Is weight control and staying in shape a constant problem?
Are you using medication or substances to make you feel better?
Have you considered ending your life?
Do you have sufficient spiritual and emotional resources?

While these questions seem to have little to do with medicine, they are intricately related to it, because they are part of the experience of my patients. What they choose to tell me in answer to these questions, or often on

their own, helps me to understand and work with their
total situation.

Common Complaints

Just as I have learned to ask certain questions of patients, so I have found that their comments often are similar. Here are some of the most common. Perhaps you have
voiced one of these yourself.

"I just don't think anyone understands my problem!"
"As a man, how could you understand what I am going
    through?"
"I've been to several doctors and have tried everything
    to solve my problem, but nothing is helping."
"I don't think that God really cares about me."
"I feel trapped in my life. I do love my family, but I feel
    as if everyone wants a part of me, and there is noth-
    ing left to give."
"Sometimes I feel as if someone or something comes
    in and takes control of my body and mind."
"It seems I spend all of my time taking care of others.
    Who is going to take care of me?"
"I wish I could quit my job, but I can't. We need the
    money, and if I don't work, the kids won't have any-
    thing to wear."
"Can I ever be forgiven for what I have done?"

As I am asked these questions, I try to give honest
answers that meet the unique needs of the questioner. Usually, my answers are rooted in the Bible; often they are
derived from something Jesus said or from some way He
interacted with women.

I realize that women feel very vulnerable when they
openly reveal not only their physical ailments but their

emotional frailties as well. They are confronting the fragile relationship between their intricate physiology and their emotions and lifestyle, between their biology and their choices. Although I do my best to help women understand the vital connection between their bodies and their way of life, I find that many of them either do not see the connection between their stresses and anxieties and the disorders that result, or they just refuse to acknowledge them when they leave the office.

God has designed and endowed you with the ability to sense and feel, to communicate and express yourself. When you sense that there is a connection between what you feel emotionally and physically, you need to deal with what is happening in all areas of your life. A doctor's prescription for pills or some advice about making lifestyle changes will not resolve your problems. You need to be willing to confront your life issues, admit their effect on you, and then devote yourself to making the changes that are needed, whether they are in diet, exercise, medication, or lifestyle, or if they involve your emotional or spiritual well-being.

How Much Does God Value You?

As you have looked into the encounters Jesus had with women, you have seen some very personal ways in which He demonstrated His special care for women, not only to heal them but to draw them to wholeness of life. These all are based on God as the Creator, the One who formed you before you were visible to others. He even wrote your name in His book as His particular creation. You may want to read Psalm 139 again. Then as you think of the miracle stories, you can know that Christ places as high a value on you as He did on women of His day, and He wants to extend the same kind of care to you.

Jesus values you enough to be concerned about your fertility. He has made the barren and the elderly able to conceive. For you, fertility may not come from your own womb, as unfair as that might seem. God may have an unwanted or unloved child born to another woman for you to nurture and raise. Be sensitive to His leading in this regard. Remember, He knows what is best for you and will enable you to accomplish it in His time.

Jesus values you enough to hear the cries you make for your children. Whether it be about illness, congenital defects, problems like attention deficit and hyperactivity disorder, or even addictions to which your child may have succumbed, remember that He loves your children even more than you do. Also, He knows what is best for them. Sometimes when they don't get what you think they need or deserve, it may turn out to be a protection and a mercy.

Jesus values you enough to go out of His way to meet your needs. Just as He detoured through Samaria for an appointment with the woman at the well (John 4:4–42), He will go to all lengths to meet you at your point of greatest need and will reach out His hand to meet that need. Don't be surprised if the manner in which He addresses you is not what you expected. He wants you to come into a personal relationship with Him, but on His terms, not yours.

Jesus values you enough to forgive you for any sin you have committed. You may think your sins are so horrendous that they can never be forgiven. But He forgave the woman caught in adultery (John 8:3–11) and Peter who denied Him (John 20:15–19). He forgave the thief on the cross (Luke 23:39–43), Zacchaeus who had cheated the poor (Luke 19:1–10), and the harlot at Simon's house (Luke 7:36–50). No matter what you have done, Jesus invites you, "Come and I will forgive." He is knocking at the door of your heart and wants you to let Him come in.

Jesus values you enough to love and support you in your grief. Just as He wept at the grave of Lazarus (John 11:33–36), Jesus weeps when He sees you suffering and grieving for the loss of a loved one or in empathy for the grief of another. In the horror of losing a child to death, He is there to comfort you and to say, "Child, I love you and I know your pain." Christ has suffered every temptation you face, and that includes the temptation to reject God when you are hurt and alienated.

Jesus values you enough to encourage you through those difficult years of menopause and older age. Just as He sensed the touch of the woman with an issue of blood (Mark 5:24–34), so He senses when you are miserable during your years of hormonal change, particularly when it seems that something comes in and takes control of your life against your will. He also knows your frailties in old age and wants to protect and comfort you.

Jesus values you enough to give His life for you. He died on the cross for you. Yes, He died for the sins of the whole world, but what really matters is that He died for you as an individual. It is a one-to-one relationship, and He reaches out to you in love and concern saying, "Come, My child, let Me love you the way you need to be loved." Only God can do that through the power of the Holy Spirit.

Meeting Jesus at the Cross

Darla came to my office on referral for an abnormal Pap smear. At twenty-eight she had already been married and divorced twice. She was currently dating a man in his late thirties. Darla's Pap smear had revealed abnormal cells in the cervix with a diagnosis of carcinoma-in-situ, which means that there were localized precancerous cells in the lining of the cervix. She had a conization done to surgically remove the outer portion of the cervix. Unfortunately, this did not completely remove all of the abnormal cells, and she required another conization.

As I worked with Darla, I realized she did not understand anything about a personal relationship with Jesus. I talked with her about her past marriages and found that she had been unfaithful to both of her husbands. As I expected, her parents had been divorced under similar circumstances. I encouraged her to start attending a singles group at a local church. There she met people who were serious about their relationship with Christ, and soon she was attending regularly.

I explained to Darla that true healing begins at the foot of the cross. There, where anyone can approach boldly, the sick find that Jesus experienced every trial that we experience today.

He experienced rejection by friends as those who had sung "Hosannas" just days before now fled. He experienced false accusations during the mock trials he endured. Verbal abuse came his way from authorities, soldiers, and people crying, "Crucify Him."

Jesus understands physical abuse from the scourging and weight of the cross on His back. He even experienced a form of sexual abuse as He was stripped of His clothing in public. He understands abandonment because Peter denied Him and John looked on from a distance.

Christ identifies even with separation from the Father because the burden of the sin of the entire world caused Him to cry out, "My God, my God, why have you forsaken me?" There is nothing that we experience that Jesus doesn't also understand personally. True healing begins at the foot of the cross.

Darla had to return to our office every three months for Pap smears, and fortunately they were all normal. During one of those visits, she said to me, "Thank you so much for introducing me to Jesus."

"Darla, I didn't introduce you to Jesus. He has been trying to introduce Himself to you for years, but you didn't hear Him. I'm just so glad that you have found peace and security in your life. Now, be sure to share your story with others—there are so many people who need Him just as you did."

Then I told her about the woman at the well. Tears streamed down her face as she said, "I'm so glad I have had my thirst quenched with that living water. It satisfies, just as He said it would!"

Notes

Chapter 2: Please Help My Child

1. Patients with anorexia nervosa often come from dysfunctional families with a social/cultural emphasis on thinness. Women with anorexia frequently give a history of extreme stress in their childhood homes. They were pushed to do or become something that they lacked the self-esteem or ability to accomplish. Just as stress can precipitate bingeing and purging, so it can stimulate a preoccupation with weight reduction to the extent that it becomes a disease. Whereas many women respond to anxiety in their lives by eating, the anorectic woman responds by doing whatever is necessary to lose weight, including starving.

Women with anorexia nervosa typically have type A personalities, have accentuated cardiovascular reactions to stress, and are perfectionistic, easily excited, and hostile with significant repressed anger. They are often very finicky and are extremely vulnerable to the mildest of stressors. They have a distorted body image, weigh less than they should, participate in eating rituals, and deny that they have a food-related problem. Anorexia is an ego-syntonic disorder, meaning that the person is proud of her emaciation.

Chapter 3: Infertility, Adoption, and Miracle Babies

1. Approximately 20 percent of infertility is male-factor and 80 percent female-factor. Most male-factor infertility is

a result of a low sperm count due to acute or chronic disease. Female-factor infertility usually results from absence of ovulation (passage of an egg from the ovary), blockage of the fallopian tubes, or other diseases that alter normal hormonal production.

2. A hysteroscope is a lighted instrument that can be placed into the uterus through the vagina to allow the use of small instruments to do procedures inside the uterus.

3. Laparoscopy is a surgical procedure in which a lighted instrument is placed into the abdominal cavity, while the patient is under general anesthesia, in order to visualize the internal structures such as the uterus, tubes, and ovaries.

4. Intrauterine insemination is a procedure in which a plastic tube is used to place the husband's sperm into the uterus at the time of ovulation; in-vitro fertilization is a method of inseminating the mother's eggs with her husband's sperm outside the body and then placing the zygote or fertilized egg into the uterus or fallopian tube.

Chapter 4: Coping with Chronic Disease

1. Debbie Warhola, "The Power of Prayer in Healing," *Colorado Springs Gazette,* 16 March 1996, Lifestyle Section, 1.

2. We are not told if the bleeding was only at the time of her menses or if it happened between her periods as well. Bleeding between periods is more frequently associated with a malignancy than is heavy bleeding at the time of the period. It is probable that she had a menstrual disorder rather than a blood-clotting problem, since she was still alive after twelve years. If her blood-clotting mechanism had been abnormal, she would likely have bled to death long before this meeting with Jesus.

3. Multiple sclerosis is a chronic, relapsing disease that involves the demyelination of neural tissue (hardening the tissue around the brain and spine). It is characterized by weakness, numbness, difficulty with coordination, balance, and gait, as well as possible visual problems.

4. Barbara Cummiskey, "The Miracle Day," *Guideposts* (April 1985), 5.

Chapter 5: *Misused Women*

1. HPV is the most frequently diagnosed sexually transmitted virus in the United States. There are many different strains of this virus, which has been recognized for centuries but only recently has become prevalent. The virus is transmitted by direct sexual contact with an infected person, and contrary to public ads and the information on condom boxes, condoms do not protect against transmission.

This viral infection progresses very slowly from initial contact to occurrence of visible lesions. The infected person may develop cauliflower-type warty lesions along with itching and pain. Many women experience no symptoms, and so they do not know they are infected until their Pap smear becomes abnormal or their sexual partner shows evidence of infection.

HPV causes 92 to 95 percent of all precancerous and cancerous lesions of the cervix. It can also cause cancer of the vulva. Treatment includes use of caustic solutions such as acetic acid, electric cautery, or laser therapy.

2. Just short of Sychar, the road to Samaria forks, and at this fork stands the well of Jacob, near a plot of land that Jacob had given to his son Joseph. This deep well was sacred to the Jews, for many memories of their people were centered there. The well was also near a mountain that the Samaritans revered—Mount Gerizim. The well is still active today, with the water table fluctuating between 75 and 105 feet. *Harper's Bible Dictionary* (San Francisco: Harper & Row, 1985), 445.

3. Chlamydia is a bacterial, sexually transmitted disease (STD) that can cause cervical infection and potentially ascend in the genital tract and infect the uterus and fallopian tubes as well, resulting in pelvic inflammatory disease, which can lead to infertility and tubal pregnancies. It is the most fre-

quent bacterial STD in the United States, infecting approximately four million persons a year. Although it can cause abnormal discharge from the vagina, most women with cervical infection are asymptomatic. Barbara had contracted a chlamydial infection and was treated with doxycycline, a type of tetracycline, and was cured of the infection.

Chapter 6: Women with Wounded Hearts

1. Pelvic inflammatory disease can result in infertility, an increased risk of tubal (ectopic) pregnancy, and chronic pelvic pain.

2. Tears, a bodily secretion with a salty composition, are produced and stored in the lacrimal glands. Tiny lacrimal ducts carry the tears to the corners of the eyes where they are released. But they aren't released until there is a reason. The reasons vary—irritation of the eye, sudden change in temperature, grief, pain in other parts of the body, sympathy for the pain or loss of another, guilt, pride of accomplishment, as well as joy and happiness.

Chapter 7: Waiting for God's Perfect Timing

1. Carole Sanderson Streeter, *Reflections for Women Alone* (Wheaton: Victor, 1987), 41–42.

2. The Apgar score is an index used to evaluate the condition of a newborn infant based on color, heart rate, reflex, muscle tone, and respiration.

3. David A. Seamands, *If Only* (Wheaton: Victor, 1995), 31–33. Used by permission.

4. Ibid., 33.

Chapter 8: Restoration for Our Children

1. *Harper's Bible Dictionary* (San Francisco: Harper & Row, 1985), 146.

2. A. Edersheim, *Sketches of Jewish Social Life* (Peabody, Mass.: Hendricksen Publishers, 1994), 154.

3. Ibid.

4. Ibid., 150–53.
5. Ibid., 156.
6. B. Witherington III, *Women and the Genesis of Christianity* (Cambridge, England: Cambridge University Press, 1990), 86.
7. James Dobson, *Life on the Edge* (Dallas: Word, 1995), 148.

Chapter 9: Jesus Cares for Senior Citizens

1. Estrogen acts on the lining of the arteries to inhibit atherosclerotic plaque deposits, which narrow and eventually block arteries that transport blood to strategic organs in the body. Some people promote the use of natural estrogens, such as wild yam extract, in order to avoid the increased risk of breast cancer associated with estrogen intake. Unfortunately, the natural estrogens have no effect on osteoporosis, coronary disease, or other physical systems helped by estrogen in pill or patch.

2. I am totally opposed to the physician-assisted suicide that is unfortunately so often in our news today. As doctors, we are in the business of helping people to live; we are not licensed to kill them. We need to effectively use the forms of pain relief we have available so that our older people can stay involved in stimulating activities. But doctors do not exist merely to hand out medicine. There are many ways we can minister to elderly patients, including spiritual and psychological prescriptions that will keep them connected to other people, as well as research toward finding ways to retard mental and emotional degeneration.

Chapter 10: What Makes the Difference in a Woman's Health?

1. D. E. King and B. Bushwick, "Beliefs and Attitudes of Hospital Inpatients about Faith Healing and Prayer," *Journal of Family Practice* 39, no. 4 (1994): 349–52.

2. Ibid.

3. T. A. Maugans and W. C. Wadland, "Religion and Family Medicine: A Survey of Physicians and Patients," *Journal of Family Practice* 32, no. 2 (1991): 210–13.

4. R. Schwab and K. U. Peterson, "Religiousness: Its Relation to Loneliness, Neuroticism, and Subjective Well-Being," *Journal for the Scientific Study of Religion* 29, no. 3 (1990): 335–45.

5. N. H. Gottlieb and L. W. Green, "Life Events, Social Network, Lifestyle, and Health: An Analysis of the 1979 National Survey of Personal Health Practices and Consequences," *Health Education Quarterly* 11 (1984): 91–105.

6. W. Sheehan and J. Kroll, "Psychiatric Patients' Belief in General Health Factors and Sin as Causes of Illness," *American Journal of Psychiatry* 147 (1990): 112–13.

7. E. P. Shafranske and H. N. Malony, "Clinical Psychologists' Religious and Spiritual Orientations and Their Practice of Psychotherapy," *Clinical Psychology* 27, no. 1 (1990): 72–78.

8. Maugans and Wadland, "Religion and Family Medicine."

9. H. J. Baltrusch, W. Stangel, and I. Titze, "Stress, Cancer and Immunity: New Developments in Biopsychosocial and Psychoneuroimmunologic Research," *Acta Neurologica* 13 (1991): 315–27.

10. Juliet Schor, *The Overworked American* (New York: Basic Books, 1992), 1–15.

11. W. D. Hager and L. C. Hager, *Stress and the Woman's Body* (Grand Rapids: Revell, 1996), 23.

12. Ibid.

13. You will find suggestions for relaxation and renewal in Hager and Hager, *Stress and the Woman's Body.*

Chapter 11: The Power of Prayer

1. Robin Marantz Henig, "Medicine's New Age," *Civilization* 4, no. 2 (April/May 1997): 42–49.

2. Marty Kaplan, "Ambushed by Spirituality," *Time,* 24 June 1996, 62.

3. Claudia Wallis, "Faith and Healing," *Time,* 24 June 1996, 60.

4. Herbert Benson, M.D., "Should You Consult Dr. God?" *Prevention* (December 1996): 62.

5. Ibid., 140.

6. Wallis, "Faith and Healing," 60.

7. Michael E. McCullough, "Prayer and Health: Conceptual Issues, Research Review, and Research Agenda," *Journal of Psychology and Theology* 25, no. 1 (1995): 16.

8. Larry Dossey, M.D., *Healing Words: The Power of Prayer and the Practice of Medicine* (San Francisco: HarperCollins, 1993), 205.

Dr. David Hager is an OB/GYN with Women's Care Center and is on the staff of the University of Kentucky Medical School. A nationally regarded expert on sexually transmitted disease, he has worked for the U.S. Centers for Disease Control in Atlanta and is on the Focus on the Family Physicians Resource Council. He and his wife, Linda, are coauthors of *Stress and the Woman's Body*. Dr. Hager also coauthored *Women at Risk*.